Therapy Over 50

Aging Issues in Psychotherapy and the Therapist's Life

Jeffrey A. Kottler

and

Jon Carlson

OXFORD
UNIVERSITY PRESS

OXFORD
UNIVERSITY PRESS

Oxford University Press is a department of the University of Oxford. It furthers the University's objective of excellence in research, scholarship, and education by publishing worldwide. Oxford is a registered trade mark of Oxford University Press in the UK and certain other countries.

Published in the United States of America by Oxford University Press
198 Madison Avenue, New York, NY 10016, United States of America.

Library of Congress Cataloging-in-Publication Data
Names: Kottler, Jeffrey A., author. | Carlson, Jon, author.
Title: Therapy over 50 : aging issues in psychotherapy and the therapist's life / Jeffrey A. Kottler and Jon Carlson.
Other titles: Therapy over fifty
Description: Oxford ; New York : Oxford University Press, [2016] |
Includes bibliographical references and index.
Identifiers: LCCN 2015036290 | ISBN 9780190205683 (alk. paper)
Subjects: LCSH: Psychotherapy for older people. | Older people—Counseling of. | Psychotherapist and patient. | Counselor and client.
Classification: LCC RC480.54 .K67 2016 | DDC 616.89/140846—dc23
LC record available at http://lccn.loc.gov/2015036290

9 8 7 6 5 4 3 2 1
Printed by Sheridan, USA

CONTENTS

PREFACE

We have written a *lot* of books about psychotherapy and counseling, many of them focused on various facets of the field, as well as some of the more personal and forbidden aspects of what it means to live and work as a helper and healer. Yet among all of our intriguing and provocative subjects about the therapist's inner experience, there is none that has been so neglected than a focus on aging issues in therapy and the therapist's life. This is a book that delves deeply into the unique challenges—and joys—of therapists who are passing into their fifth decade and beyond.

This is a book intended for practitioners (and students) within the various helping professions, including social work, psychology, psychiatry, family therapy, mental health counseling, pastoral counseling, and addictions therapy. It is especially targeted for any clinicians who work with older clients—or those who aspire to do so—which should be almost everyone. In addition, we also address many of the issues most relevant to older therapists (or those who are growing older) who have an interest in learning more about the implications and consequences of their growth, development, and biological changes. Just as intriguing are the ways that cultural pressures influence the aged to make certain adaptations to the ways they work and live, not to mention the ways we all view ourselves.

According to surveys conducted by various professional organizations within counseling and psychotherapy, the average age of a practitioner is in the mid 50s (Michalski & Kohut, 2008; National Association of Social Workers, 2006; Scully & Wilk, 2003). When we add to that figure the legions of those on the cusp of "senior" status, we can readily appreciate that aging is a central component of all professional development, but especially so for those of us who specialize in change for a living.

If growing older is a reality of life in our profession, with all its accompanying adaptations, then it is even more of a significant issue for our clients in an aging culture. It is expected that by the year 2030, as many as 20% of the U.S. population will be older than 65 years (Administration on Aging, 2011), compared with less than 8% in 1950. On a worldwide scale, during the next four decades, the number of people 85 years and older will be five times greater than it is now (Laidlaw & Pachana, 2009). This means that, for most therapists, older clients may represent a tiny percentage of their caseload; in the future, however, they may very well comprise the bulk of those who are referred. As never before, older people have more discretionary time, more resources, and more willingness to delve into matters of emotional well-being.

Although the age of 50 is no longer considered to be "old," at least compared with the life expectancies of previous centuries, it is still often considered an artificial boundary that signals another phase in life characterized by a different set of challenges. This is the stage in life that Erik Erikson described as the beginning of generativity, when our life's mission transforms into a role designed to mentor and nurture others if we wish to avoid stagnation and despair. It is a time within middle age to take stock of our life's work and make new choices about how to use the limited time we have left.

For our increasingly aging clients, psychotherapy becomes a place to talk about the inevitable and unrelenting changes that are taking place, as well as to come to terms with lost dreams. Changes in hormones and metabolism, muscle mass and bone density, sensory acuity, energy levels, sleep patterns, sexual responsiveness, family roles, cultural status, as well as self-identity and expectations by others, produce all kinds of disequilibrium that often require considerable adjustments. The willingness and ability to adapt to changes, as well as to continue new learning and growth, are absolutely essential for life satisfaction during the latter part of life (Hill, 2005). Psychotherapy can—and should be—a useful, if not necessary, part of that continued learning and growth.

It isn't just the ways that older people feel differently than they did in their youth, but also how they are *treated* differently by others.

"I used to be someone important," one woman in her 60s said with a shrug. "I ran my division with more than 70 staff reporting to me. We had among the highest profitability in. . . ." She paused with a sad kind of smile, momentarily lost in a memory, then shook her head and flicked her hand as if brushing off an annoying, persistent insect. "It's just that . . . I don't know . . . I used to be someone who others listened to, who they respected. But ever since I retired I feel invisible. Even people who used to pay attention to me, who seemed to value what I had to say, now seem to ignore me. Or even worse, it feels like they are merely indulging me to be polite."

It is clear that older people have unique problems and different worldviews than those that were commonplace during the early stages of the profession, when the focus was on helping bored and disillusioned Victorian women, children with learning difficulties, and returning veterans from the First World War. The counseling profession, for example, was originally developed to address the needs of the school-age population. Much of the research in psychology has relied primarily on studying relatively healthy, successful college students—the most accessible subjects for academics. All the early and classic textbooks on human development devoted most of the attention to the first two decades of life, when all the action supposedly takes place, adding a few feeble sections at the end to the last decades of existence. It was as if nothing much interesting happens after adolescence except the long, slow slog toward deterioration and death.

Yet, today's clientele are so different as the various helping professions have matured and evolved—and most of us have been singularly unprepared to adapt what we do, and how we do it, to meet more effectively the needs of people struggling with very different issues than the ones discussed traditionally in the literature. Just as interesting—and imperative—are the ways therapists over 50 have learned (or been required) to work very differently as a result of aging. Issues related to diminished memory, fatigue, and bladder control, as well as quite different family and professional contexts, require a number of adaptations.

Aging clients often feel as though they are mostly placated by others, even by their therapists, and are being put out to pasture when they are more likely just hitting their stride and finally locating aspects of themselves for which they have been searching for a lifetime. Beginning therapists, however well meaning, often share the same biases of our culture, which worships youth in a multitude of ways. They may resent their older colleagues who are standing in their way and inadvertently treat their older clients with less respect and compassion than they deserve. Older clients want to be understood for who they really are despite repeated messages they receive that they are over the hill and incapable of living a satisfying life.

What we find most ironic and incomprehensible about this topic is how little interest many practitioners express in learning more about this specialty area although it is—and will become—such a critical part of therapeutic expertise. Although this observation is based on a limited sample, we couldn't help but notice how reluctant and resistant many of our colleagues were to talk about their aging challenges. Although in many of our previous projects our response rate for invitations to contribute insights was close to 75% or more, we found that only a very few notable theorists were willing to participate in this project. When we were investigating failures (Kottler & Carlson, 2002), unusual cases (Kottler & Carlson, 2003), reciprocal influence (Kottler & Carlson, 2006), spiritual transformations (Kottler & Carlson, 2007), best sessions (Kottler & Carlson, 2008), advocacy and social justice (Kottler & Marriner, 2009; Kottler, Englar-Carlson, & Carlson, 2013), creative breakthroughs (Kottler & Carlson, 2009), deceit and lying in therapy (Kottler, 2010; Kottler & Carlson, 2011), and therapeutic mastery (Kottler & Carlson, 2015), prominent therapists were practically begging us to talk to them about their experiences. Let's just say that it took considerable persistence and effort to find a similar group of distinguished therapists to talk about what it means to deal with aging issues as they come up in sessions and in their own lives. And this isn't just unique to our profession. Most doctors, as well, are relatively clueless about the challenges related to aging because only 3% have ever had any training in gerontology (Gawande, 2014).

Is this denial? Are we so apprehensive about talking about growing old that we prefer to keep the subject at arm's length? It would certainly seem so considering that most books published on the subject offer cheerful, optimistic promises in their titles such as *Positive Aging, Optimal Aging, The Sexy Years,* and *Younger Next Year.* Our relative ignorance is compounded by the assumption that as we grow older ourselves, that qualifies us as experts on the subject.

Although therapists routinely receive training in child therapy, play therapy, adolescent therapy, couples therapy, family therapy, sex therapy, and other clinical specialties, it is rare that programs offer required courses in working with the elderly. Although almost all therapists see older clients at some time, less than 3% have ever actually received any training with this group (Kraus, 2012). This means there has been little preparation for dealing with the unique challenges of these clients, including their declining health, mortality, and existential issues related to spirituality, isolation, losses, and meaning making (Suri, 2010). Even more perplexing is how unpopular most books on this subject are compared with other topics. Perhaps this isn't all that surprising considering that, many years ago, a study confirmed what is easy to surmise—that therapists much prefer seeing younger clients and don't like to see older ones because of a perception that their prognoses are too poor and their patterns too entrenched to be altered (Zivian, Larsen, Knox, Gekoski, & Hatchette, 1992). Given the demographic certainty that working with the aged will become the greatest need for the future of our profession, it is about time we addressed the salient issues most relevant for this population, as well as those for the more than half of therapists who are over 50.

CONTENTS OF THE BOOK

Because there is often a parallel process operating during sessions in which both clients and therapists are reflecting and personalizing what is taking place, it seems logical that we would discuss aging issues as they might affect all participants. Certainly this includes transference, countertransference, and projective identification phenomena, but, far more than that, there are just so many interesting—and largely ignored—issues that arise that could make us so much more effective in our work, as well as personally satisfied.

We explore the experience of aging in therapy from two different sides. The first theme looks at how therapists over 50, or those approaching that life transition, experience, struggle, and enjoy doing therapy in ways that are different from when they were younger. This includes their special challenges and adaptations, their fears and their joys. Second, we cover the landscape related to working clinically with aging clients, specifically those approaches and strategies that work best with this population. Both of these topics, although seemingly covering very different material, are actually integrally related because of the nature of reciprocal influence in helping relationships. Although we include both current research and classic literature on the subject of aging issues in therapy, we have also gained access to some notable aging figures in the field, and have interviewed dozens of older clients and therapists who have some clear thoughts on what aging means to them, for better or worse (mostly for the better).

We begin with an introduction, discussing what led us to this subject that we have both avoided—until such time we seemed to have no choice in the matter. Like so many of our research projects, this one was conceived out of personal adversity and confusion. The introduction is followed by the first chapter, which covers what it means to be older and the various ways that aging is defined and experienced. Continuing the first section of the book about aging in personal and professional development, Chapter 2 explores the ways that identity is shaped and influenced by culture, and the scripts that people learn about what it means to be old.

The second part of the book looks at aging within the life and practice of the therapist. What does it mean to be an "elder" or senior practitioner in the field (Chapter 3)? Although Chapter 4 talks about some of the biological realities of aging, both the physical challenges as well as distinct advantages, Chapter 5 focuses more specifically on "tricks of the trade" that usually occur for more experienced practitioners. Chapter 6 follows this theme by discussing the accumulation of wisdom in a life's work.

In the third part of the book, we move from a discussion of the therapist's experience of aging to the salient clinical issues for older clients. We start with some of the myths and misconceptions about aging (Chapter 7), as well as the some of the challenges that are often faced (Chapters 8 and 9). Chapters 10 and 11 highlight some of the specialized therapeutic strategies designed for working with aging clients, and some of the most effective adaptations that experts make to produce better outcomes. In one sense, this isn't all that different from what we do to alter our style and approach with a client from *any* distinct "cultural" group, although there are indeed some unique considerations to keep in mind. Chapter 12 discusses a subject that clients (and therapists) would most like to avoid, and that is the impending prospect of failing health and death. The last chapter speaks honestly about the dreams that are lost with aging, as well as new aspirations that are just as fulfilling.

ACKNOWLEDGMENTS

In many ways, this has been our most challenging book to write. Not only is the breadth and depth of the subject so big, but also it is about one of those subjects that evoke discomfort, if not terror, in many people who feel a certain reluctance and ambivalence in talking about what it means to be old. As with so many of our other projects, our editor, Dana Bliss, was a constant fountain of support and encouragement. Several times we attempted to abandon this project because of the difficult issues it stirred up for us, but Dana insisted we persevere.

We are also appreciative to a number of the individuals who agreed to speak with us about their own experiences related to aging processes, especially Marianne Corey, Jerry Englar, Howard Kirschenbaum, Michael Hoyt, Claudia Black, Nicholas Cummings, Jerry Corey, Ann Vernon, Pat Love, Rosanne Tadsen, Phil Kirk, Leita Englar, Don Ardell, Catherine Jenni, and Hank Sibbing.

Jeffrey A. Kottler
Huntington Beach, California

Jon Carlson
Lake Geneva, Wisconsin, and Chicago, Illinois

ABOUT THE AUTHORS

This book is written by two therapists who have struggled with a host of challenges related to aging, including diagnoses of cancer and failing health, significant physical decline, disrupted sleep problems, decreased memory and energy, as well as serious existential crises related to impending death and the ongoing search for meaning. In addition, they have managed to demonstrate extraordinary resilience, flexibility, creativity, and courage in facing a number of life challenges, accumulating 80 years of clinical experience and authoring 100 books between them. Despite a number of difficulties and obstacles, they managed to reinvent themselves and remain continually energized and passionate about their work, reaching a stage in life in which they have (almost) embraced their role as wise elders.

Jeffrey A. Kottler, PhD, is one of the most prolific authors in the fields of psychology and education, having written more than 80 books about a wide range of subjects during the past 40 years. He has authored more than a dozen texts for counselors and therapists that are used in universities around the world, and dozens of books for practicing therapists and educators. Some of his previous titles include *On Being a Therapist, The Compleat Therapist, Travel That Can Change Your Life, Creative Breakthroughs in Therapy: Tales of Transformation and Astonishment, The Therapist's Workbook: Self-assessment, Self-care, and Self-improvement Exercises for Mental Health Professionals, Learning Group Leadership, The Assassin and the Therapist: An Exploration of Truth in Psychotherapy and in Life, Changing People's Lives while Transforming Your Own: Paths to Social Justice and Global Human Rights, Divine Madness: Ten Stories of Creative Struggle, Change: What Leads to Personal Transformation, Stories We've Heard, Stories We've Told: Life-Changing Narratives in Therapy and Everyday Life,* and *The Therapist in the Real World: What You Never Learn in Graduate School (But Really Need to Know).*

Jeffrey has worked as a teacher, counselor, and therapist in a preschool, middle school, mental health center, crisis center, university, community college, and private-practice settings. He has served as a Fulbright scholar in Peru (1980) and Iceland (2000), as well as worked as a visiting professor in New Zealand, Australia, Hong Kong, Singapore, and Nepal. Jeffrey is professor of counseling at California State University, Fullerton; and founder of Empower Nepali Girls, an organization that provides educational scholarships for at-risk children in Nepal and provides medical and trauma services to survivors of the 2015 earthquakes.

Jon Carlson, PsyD, EdD, spent much of his career as distinguished professor of psychology and counseling at Governors State University, University Park, Illinois; and as a psychologist with the Wellness Clinic in Lake Geneva, Wisconsin. He is currently a distinguished professor of Adlerian Psychology at Adler University in Chicago. He spends much of his time doing live demonstrations of therapy and conducting workshops around the world, most recently in Thailand, Lithuania, and Romania.

Jon is the author of 60 books covering many facets of psychotherapy, family therapy, marital enrichment, consultation, loneliness, and Adlerian psychology. Some of his best known works include *How Master Therapists Work, Adlerian Therapy, Never Be Lonely Again, Creating Connection, Love Intimacy and the African American Couple, Inclusive Cultural Empathy,* and *Time for a Better Marriage.* Jon has also produced 300 video programs that feature the most prominent leaders in the field demonstrating their theories in action. These videos are used to train the next generation of practitioners. He has received lifetime achievement awards from several professional associations, including the American Psychological Association and the American Counseling Association.

Together, Jeffrey and Jon have collaborated on several other books, including *Bad Therapy, The Mummy at the Dining Room Table, The Client Who Changed Me, American Shaman, Their Finest Hour, Moved By the Spirit, Creative Breakthroughs in Therapy, Duped: Lies and Deception in Psychotherapy, Helping Beyond the 50-Minute Hour: Therapists Involved in Meaningful Social Action,* as well as *On Being a Master Therapist: Practicing What We Preach.*

Most recently Jon is learning to enjoy disengagement from professional work, and has invited Jeffrey to join him at his cabin in northern Wisconsin where they are most likely planning their next book project.

Therapy Over 50

PART I

Aging in Personal and Professional Development

CHAPTER 1
What It Means to Be Older

"As we get older, and I've learned it as I've aged, I don't quite heal as fast as I used to. I just don't bounce back like I used to. That's just part of aging."

This man is complaining about the ravaging effects of growing older, resulting in chronic pain and significant limits on his physical abilities. His performance in a number of areas that matter most to him have diminished significantly and he wonders if he will ever regain full functioning again. He was also only 37 years old—and the speaker is professional golfer Tiger Woods, who is talking about how aware he has become of his limitations: he's not the person he used to be and he's not yet hit 40.

In this chapter we address some of the central issues that affect and define what it means to grow older. As we are quite aware, developmental experiences are shaped not only by biological factors, but also by social influences that lead to particular self-perceptions. This is true not the larger community and within the culture of mental health professionals.

THE INVENTION OF OLD AGE

Old age is a relatively new phenomenon among our species and a rather new specialty area among mental health professionals. G. Stanley Hall, one of the pioneers in developing psychology as a discipline distinct from philosophy, was also among the first to study the adjustment challenges of aging systematically. For all practical purposes, old age, as a universal phenomenon, didn't even exist until the latter part of the 19th century, when Hall was conducting his early research on human development.

As one of the founders of gerontology, Hall warned that with longer life spans, limited employment opportunities, and changing roles within the family, there was increasing danger that older people would become increasingly isolated. Hall became aware of how these forces impacted his own life as he grew older, and he was considered a prophet in predicting that the plight of the elderly would only grow worse over time. Among his many accomplishments as the first professor of psychology, distinguished scholar of genetic and psychophysiological psychology, president of a university, and responsible for first inviting Sigmund Freud to lecture in America, Hall also became a passionate spokesperson against the stigma of aging.

It is certainly understandable how staggeringly rapid changes in human evolution related to life span would catch the dominant culture by surprise. What is a community to do with individuals who are past childbearing age, are no longer able to hunt or gather food as effectively as in their youth, and are often a drain on limited resources? Within other species of living creatures, time expires when individuals are no longer "useful" they are required to make room for the young and fertile. There are other reasons, as well, for valuing youth over age in that time takes a toll on cellular functioning—creating molecular disruptions, vulnerability to disease, and compromised condition. Genetic programming is designed in such a way that metabolic functioning gradually slows down until the clock winds down and cells are regenerated and reborn in other forms so they can get a fresh start. What has happened with human evolution is both unprecedented and poorly understood.

For so many thousands of years of our existence, human beings were fortunate to survive until their 20s. Most infants died before their first year, along with a rate of maternal mortality that was staggering. Even as late as the beginning of the 20th century, one-quarter of all children died before the age of five. And then, virtually overnight, or at least within the span of several decades, infant and maternal mortality were reduced by more than 90% (Carstensen, 2011; Francis, 2002). For the first time in human history, it was not only possible, but also likely that those who had access to reasonable nutrition and healthcare could live many decades longer. It may take evolution tens of thousands of years to alter physiology, but it took only a single generation for cultural adaptations and modern science to extend life well into the 80s and beyond.

There are currently more Americans older than 85 than there are teenagers. There are soon expected to be more elderly Chinese (300 million) than there are people in the United States. Because of reduced birth rates, better medical care, improved diet, and increased longevity, the elderly are the fastest growing segment of the world population (Cruikshank, 2009). In Japan, sales of adult diapers now exceed those for infants, which may be one reason why one Japanese political figure, the finance minister, recommended the elderly be shipped off to nursing homes in the Philippines (Pilling, 2003).

This brings us to one of the puzzling scientific questions regarding why Nature even "allows" older people to continue to exist, considering they have ceased to serve the primary biological imperative of propagating our species. At first glance, they seem to be a drain on the community, no longer contributing to the productive workforce, especially during ancient times of famine and limited food sources. What good are the elderly if they can no longer operate at peak performance, no longer reproduce, take up valuable space and resources, and often represent a burden?

The obvious answer, connected integrally to the therapist's primary professional role, is that the elderly are essentially storage facilities that hold accumulated knowledge useful to others in the community. They are the holders and disseminators of wisdom. They know the locations of the best hunting grounds and water holes. They know the most expeditious routes across geographic obstacles. They are familiar with other tribal groups that inhabit the same territory. And as a function of their life experiences, they recognize patterns and can solve problems they have encountered previously. They are also more likely to make altruistic choices that are advantageous for the community than for their own selfish interests.

This leads to one other explanation for why Nature has permitted older human beings to exist: evolving another strategy to ensure survival of the larger community. Among many other species—bottlenose dolphins, killer whales, Seychelles warblers—the presence of older adults increases the likelihood that offspring will survive with the added assistance of members who are beyond childbearing years. This is also the case with respect to human beings in that the presence of older females, in particular, increases the likelihood that grandchildren will survive (Jeste & Oswald, 2014).

WHAT IS AGING ANYWAY?

A number of researchers and philosophers have been wondering why we age at all. Is this part of some grand evolutionary scheme to make room for subsequent generations? Is aging just about accumulative wear and tear, like some complex machine that eventually stops working when critical parts fail?

It used to be assumed that our longevity was predetermined genetically, based on the life span of parents. Although it may be true that our eventual height is 90% determined by what we inherited from our parents, it turns out that only a miniscule factor (6%) of parental longevity actually affects how long we will live (Vaupel, 2010).

Strictly speaking, aging is a cellular phenomenon that results from a kind of molecular clock that winds down through a process of erosion. Cells can only divide themselves and reproduce a finite number of times before they start breaking down or falling apart. Over time, they develop toxic conditions that, in the language of biology, become "free radicals" as the result of accumulations of abnormal binding in "glycation," and reduced amounts of growth hormones and too many glucocorticoid stress hormones (Butler, 2008). As far as neurons in the brain, we lose as many as three-quarters of the cells by age 70 to 90, especially in areas that control memory and emotional regulation. In other words, cells begin to lose their structural and functional ability to clear out toxins and recover from normal activity.

Despite the inevitable physiological changes that take place, life experience and accumulated expertise more than make up for the losses. The aging brain does not so much become weaker as it adapts to erosion of synaptic connections and depletion of neurotransmitters as it becomes *different*, acting less as a problem solver of novel challenges as it operates primarily in pattern recognition (Goldberg, 2005). This reframing and reformulation of what it means to age alters the dominant cultural script such that those in the last chapters of their lives are not "retired" or "put out to pasture," but rather serve a crucial survival function for humanity to provide continuity and collective knowledge. It is our job to help people celebrate and honor this important role.

WHAT QUALIFIES AS OLD?

Is age a biological condition or state of mind? We have known people in their 40s who talk constantly about how old they feel, and others in their 80s who report never feeling more vital and engaged with life. There is, therefore, considerable debate regarding when someone becomes "old," or when this stage of life begins. Depending on geographic location, ethnicity, gender, era, and even profession, being old has very different meanings. The average life expectancy for a coal miner during the early part of the 20th century was about 45 years; reaching 40 was considered a milestone. Other definitions mark this stage of life beginning at 50, 55, 62, 65, and, more recently, considerably beyond those figures.

Technically and literally, you are "over the hill" when you hit age 37, the age at which you are older than the majority of the people in the United States. In general, however, old age is considered to begin between 60 and 65, when most people start noticing more significant changes in cognitive and physical functioning (Stuart-Hamilton, 2012), although a consensus based on public opinion is that old age begins at 68, even though only 20% of people that age say they actually *feel* old (Taylor, 2009). Because the life span has expanded so much further during the past 50 years, and individual differences are so great in terms of how aging is experienced, many gerontologists have now subdivided this stage of life into "young-old" (60–69 years), "middle-aged old" (70–79), "old-old" (80–89), and the "really, really, really old" (90+ years). Yet, if "old" has generally been conceptualized as the last decade before the average life span, then age 60 really is the new middle age and oldness really doesn't begin until the middle 70s.

In addition, age can be considered somewhat arbitrarily as a chronological number or in more functional terms of how someone actually operates in the world. After all, there are potentially huge differences between how any two 70-year-olds might function, just as there are quite different issues and challenges faced by a 65-year-old versus a 95-year-old. This means that therapists have to be very careful in their assessments of clients based on chronological age that may not be a very useful predictor of actual functioning (Laidlaw & Pachana, 2009).

Likewise, self-perceptions of aging are very much a subjective experience, influenced by the ways others respond, as well as experiences within the body. One woman in her 70s, herself a therapist, describes her own sudden awareness of this phenomenon.

"I knew getting old would happen at some time, but just not yet. I just didn't think about it. I was surprised when I was faced with the reality of being an 'older adult,' and I was somewhat shocked and very humbled." She shakes her head in wonderment, remembering a particular moment of revelation: "The reality set in when I looked in the mirror one day and this old person looked back at me. I didn't want to recognize this image. Another time, when I made a motion to get my driver's license out and prove that I could get a senior discount, the clerk told me not to bother. 'I believe you,' she said!"

This therapist also realized the aging process had caught up with her when she would ask her body to do things that it was no longer willing to comply. "It has taken some time to come to terms with getting old, yet as my mother-in-law would say, 'I am over 90 years old but I have very young feelings inside.'"

Biologically speaking, aging is defined as the slow, gradual, and time-dependent process of deterioration that occurs after reproductive maturation as a result of reduced energy available for cellular division. It is both inevitable and irreversible. Regardless of one's actual age, this stage of life is usually thought to begin at the point when someone is no longer sexually active, experiences memory problems, or retires from meaningful employment.

THE THIRD CHAPTER

However "old" is defined operationally, and at what age it is supposed to begin, it is generally agreed that this stage of life is now quite long, extending multiple decades. It is a time of losses on multiple levels, and almost certain adjustments and adaptations. It is a period when people are released from previous roles and responsibilities, whether raising a family or producing prodigious quantities of work. Yet with these altered conditions, it is an era of more personal discretionary time, when options for the future become more limited. It is thus a period of reinvention, even as negative stereotypes frequently cast disparaging images of growing old as almost a crime.

The years between 50 and 65 have been described as "the third chapter of life," a period of adaptation and exploration with all kinds of possibilities for creativity and adventure (Lawrence-Lightfoot, 2009). Just as during the past century adolescence was identified and defined as a distinct developmental period, so, too, is the third chapter of life evolving as a new stage characterized by unique challenges and opportunities.

There has been so much study of the necessary developmental tasks of childhood—those progressive skills that build on one another to ensure successful adaptation and growth. For instance, children are expected to crawl, walk, and talk by a particular age, just as they must master various cognitive, emotional, and moral keystones. For the aging adult, there are also some crucial tasks that must (or should) be tackled if one is to attain some kind of fulfillment, if not enlightenment. In writing about her journey as an aging therapist, Loeb (2009) included a personal list of the developmental milestones she found most significant to navigate during her 60s. Although some of the tasks would be expected, such as coming to terms with the inevitability of death, accepting the physical changes that take place with aging, navigating an increasingly interdependent role, others delved far more deeply into existential issues, which involved the following accomplishments:

- Accepting imperfections and mistakes in yourself and others; letting go of past disappointments and failures
- Healing and repairing relationships that have been less than ideal; practicing forgiveness
- Mourning losses and disappointments that still have a hold; honoring the wounds as a kind of noble suffering
- Challenging feelings of envy toward others and, instead, accessing feelings of gratitude for what you do have
- Constructing new, realistic goals for creativity and productivity
- Discovering alternative sources of comfort and satisfaction as obsolete coping strategies are necessarily abandoned
- Accessing greater internal sources of soothing and comfort to maintain a degree of self-control and independence

The main issue with which Loeb struggled during this major life transition was whether to do less or more.

"When I was 60," she admitted, "my most immediate source of unhappiness was the disparity between my lifelong goals and the reality of my accomplishments" (Loeb, 2009, p. 188). This is what Erik Erikson and other developmental theorists mean when they talk about finding renewed meaning in a different kind of productivity and accomplishment, as well as coming to accept the dreams and desires that will never be fulfilled.

Loeb's sense of self, her very self-esteem, had been compromised because of some disappointments. This required a grieving process as well as self-forgiveness for being less than her ideal. There was no crime committed just because she didn't reach her perfect potential: "I felt successful as a psychologist, as a teacher, as a mother, but I had other dreams, other ambitious that were now no longer possible" (p. 188).

Resolution of these issues arrived for her, not through honoring past accomplishments or dwelling on ways she fell short, but rather by focusing a lot less on external sources of validation and a lot more on internal sources of satisfaction. Eventually this led to a kind of "second adulthood," a redefined identity that led to a new sense of who she was and what was still within her grasp.

THE OPPRESSION AND MARGINALIZATION OF ELDERS

Free associate "old person" and the images that come to mind are usually less than flattering. Some of the most common descriptors might include frumpy, disabled, lonely, isolated, shriveled, bitter, geezer, grouchy, forgetful, demanding, conservative, helpless, frail, and so many other negative connotations. Some of the most common myths associated with the elderly (and they are indeed misconceptions) include that most of them are senile, rigid, and unproductive, and basically stop learning (Tan, 2011). In fact, as we grow older there is even *greater* diversity in ability, interests, and levels of functioning. As never before, many people in their 80s and beyond remain remarkably active and productive, involved in a variety of advocacy and social justice causes, leadership positions in the community, political activism, and caregiving assignments (Wiles & Jayasinha, 2013).

Ageism has become so pervasive in our culture that it is no longer noticed, much less challenged the way we would confront overt racism, gender inequality, or even homophobia. In surveys of people older than 60, one-third reported experiences of being ignored or not taken seriously, and 80% said they frequently encountered others who assumed they were impaired or had memory problems because of their older appearance—so-called "senior moments" (Dittman, 2003). In another study, two-thirds of older individuals were the butt of demeaning jokes that made fun of them (Palmore, 2001). Two examples illustrate the tone of this humor.

An older woman stopped me on the street to ask me to show her how to get to the nearest hospital. So I pushed her under a bus.

Two older men in a retirement village were hanging out in the leisure room talking about their lives. "So," the younger of the two asked his friend, "how do you really feel? Honestly, you are approaching your 70th birthday; how do you feel?"

"Honestly?" he replied. "I feel like a newborn baby."
"Really?"
"Sure. I've got no hair, no teeth, and I just wet myself."

The derogatory names attributed to older people are just as inappropriate, even scandalous: old biddy, old goat, old fart, old bat, hag, old bag, geezer, codger, fossil, old fogey, battle axe, has-been, fuddy-duddy, coot, dinosaur, blue-hair, to mention just a few. Further indignities toward the aged take place when they are herded into "ghettos" called "old folks homes" (usually sanitized as "retirement communities" or "assisted-living facilities"), isolated from the general community where they might make others uncomfortable shuffling along at a leisurely pace. Even when older people choose such living arrangements it is often because they don't wish to be a burden on their families. On the other hand, they may also wish to hang out with "their own kind." Leisure World, a retirement community in southern California, incorporated itself as an actual municipality with its own mayor and city council.

Public media have not been exactly kind in their portrayal of older people, often presenting them as feeble-minded, forgetful characters, sometimes lovable, and often crotchety and cantankerous. Stories in the news often show them as helpless victims. When they appear at all in television or films, they often play foolish roles or peripheral characters rarely acting heroically.

There is a movement afoot among journalists to ban the terms *elderly* or *senior citizens* as offensive and instead refer to *older adults*. The point is to become more aware of the ways our language usage only reinforces their diminished status. This is even the case with respect to health professionals who may see the elderly as impervious to change and hardly worth the effort to attempt therapeutic or medical interventions. Emergency room physicians, frustrated with chronically ill older patients who don't respond to their immediate efforts, sometimes refer to them as "crocks," "turkeys," "dirtballs," "hateful," GOMERS (Get out of My Emergency Room), or LOLINAD (Little Old Lady in No Apparent Distress). Each of these names reflect the sense of helplessness that health professionals feel when attempting to treat intractable conditions that don't improve. In addition, they represent a dehumanizing and distancing phenomenon common in conditions of extreme stress. This is highlighted in one comment by a young doctor. "To me, a patient in the ER at 3 a.m. with a needle broken off in his neck calling me a 'motherfucker' is a dirtball. That's the way I feel about him or her and hence I may as well use the term" (Dans, 2002, p. 28).

This physician insists that the patient's care would in no way be compromised.

This situation also seems to reflect the inadequate resources available for older adults. Many visit doctors, or even call emergency services, as a means of connecting with other humans. One therapist volunteered to work with a local emergency response team to provide training in counseling skills. In preparation for the event, he studied posttraumatic stress disorder and some of the other documented problems from trauma that emergency personnel frequently encounter. When the therapist asked emergency personnel what they wanted to talk about, without hesitation they immediately requested help on how to handle the "emergency calls" from lonely residents who just wanted some attention and someone to talk to. This stunned the emergency personnel, who had no idea—like most of the larger population—how important it is to feel connected to others, especially by those who have been most marginalized and neglected.

Several studies have highlighted that negative attitudes toward the elderly are still quite prevalent among mental health practitioners, especially among those who are younger and just beginning their careers (Chonody, Webb, Ranzjin, & Bryan, 2014; Lun, 2011; Van Dussen & Weaver, 2009). Many therapists and physicians also believe that depression, and even suicidal thoughts, are simply normal and acceptable for older people, although the incidence of these symptoms is no greater than for younger people (Brody, 2007). Yet, depression is also often underdiagnosed for older clients because of an assumption often made by mental health professionals that it just comes with the territory.

As we discuss throughout the book, many professionals approach the elderly and their problems with a "Why bother?" attitude because they are going to die soon anyway. Many of today's therapists have been trained to save people and to help them return to fully functioning and productive living. With many of their elderly clients, this is not possible, leaving the therapist to feel helpless and discouraged. After all, who among us got into this field because we dreamed of helping people merely cope with their problems instead of overcoming them? Without proper training and understanding of the aging population, many therapists may avoid or serve their needs badly.

Just as serious are the relatively common instances of older people, some as young as 50, who remain unemployed or underemployed because of age discrimination. Although members of Congress and the Supreme Court can—and do—serve well into their 80s, states have been allowed, even encouraged, to discriminate on the basis of age (Gullette, 2011). With the economic downturn, adult children moving back home, and loss of retirement benefits, many older people are forced to return to work although they are frequently discouraged by limited opportunities.

Equally distressing are the ways that older people are far more likely to lack adequate healthcare services. This is no more clearly evident than during disasters such as 9/11 or the floods of New Orleans in 2005. After the fall of the Twin Towers in New York, pets were evacuated almost immediately, or within 24 hours of the attack, yet older people who had been disabled or were isolated in their homes waited more than a week for rescue or for the restoration of basic services and care (Butler, 2008). In the case of New Orleans, although 12% of the population was older than 65 at the time of the flood, close to three-quarters of all those who perished were elderly (Kahanna, 2005). It is clear that in so many ways our culture not only marginalizes older people supposedly in their "golden years," but also considers them utterly disposable.

Still more disturbing are the ways that longevity is compromised by these negative stereotypes. In one groundbreaking, longitudinal study, it was found that those who had an optimistic and resilient attitude toward growing older actually lived more than seven years longer than those who held the dominant culture's largely negative views (Levy, Slade, Kunkel, & Kasl, 2002). In addition, older people with debilitating injuries or diseases who hold positive attitudes toward their age and stations in life are far more likely to make a full recovery (Levy, Slade, Murphy, & Gill, 2012). As in so many other aspects of life, internalized scripts and cognitive interpretations of experience often influence, if not determine, what we become. Depression, anxiety, and other emotional problems may be caused as much by cultural indoctrination as any biological or psychological condition.

BIASES AND PREJUDICES AMONG HEALTH PROFESSIONALS

We discussed earlier how health professionals share many of the negative attitudes toward the elderly, joining a collective cultural conspiracy to keep older people sedated and shelved out of the way (Gomberg, 1996). Many health professionals, therapists among them, may feel a certain reluctance, if not ambivalence, working with elderly patients for all sorts of reasons we have mentioned: (a) they often present intractable, chronic conditions that are only going to get worse over time; (b) the professional's own sense of helplessness and incompetence are triggered by feeling unable to "fix" the presenting problems; and (c) one's own fears of deterioration and death are triggered as a result of intimate contact with those who are perceived as falling apart (Langle & Probst, 2000). Rather than celebrating aging, it is most often denied, disguised, or literally colored, dewrinkled, and surgically altered.

Yet in other surveys that ask people their impressions of older adults, there are also images of tranquility, maturity, wisdom, balance, experience, dependability, warmth, and caring (Lyons, 2009). These perceptions of aging are strongly influenced by the particular age of the respondent; younger people perceive the elderly far more negatively than those who older (Musaiger & D'Souza, 2009). Moreover, younger therapists are hardly exempt from these perceptions, holding their own fears and apprehensions about what it means to be old (Laidlaw & Pachana, 2009).

The roles, functions, and goals of psychotherapy will continue to evolve in coming years, paralleling the changes in the human life cycle. With a significant portion of the population likely to enjoy, or at least capture, 20, 30, or more years beyond so-called retirement, often in good health and without work or other major responsibilities, there will be an increasing need to help people clarify goals and desires for the future (Gilleard & Higgs, 2007). More and more, the question that will be addressed in sessions is: "Who and what shall I become in this next phase of life?" In that sense, older clients will become the next best ideal candidates for what we do in therapy.

IDEAL CANDIDATES FOR THERAPY

Although, traditionally, older people have pretty much been written off as legitimate participants in therapy, they are actually ideal clients in many ways. In one sense they have a greater capacity for insight because they've had more opportunities for reflection. They also have more available time to attend sessions regularly and to follow through on commitments that have been discussed. They reflect deeply on what was discussed during the therapy sessions and they come to follow-up sessions prepared and willing to participate actively. They are also often highly motivated to make sense of their lives and integrate life experiences, as well as to plan for the final stage that lies ahead.

Although many will make the pilgrimage to therapy for inspiration, enlightenment, or reflection on their life journey, others are more concerned with addressing some very real fears, worries, and challenges that few others may understand.

> *Will I lose my mind?* Anyone older than 50 has noticed cognitive changes related to memory and retrieval of information. After age 65, those changes become far more noticeable, producing almost daily occurrences when you forget a friend's name or walk into a room and can't recall what you're looking for. Although Alzheimer's disease is hardly inevitable, some selective loss of mental ability is certain. For many people, these changes are only minor inconveniences because of adaptations that take place. Therapy can and does help, not only to offer support and reassurance, but also to help with necessary adaptations.
>
> *Will my money last?* This is a fairly legitimate fear considering that income is down and expenses continue to increase with medical care, prescriptions, long-term care, and cost of living. With so-called entitlements and social security in potential jeopardy, fears are magnified further.
>
> *Will I lose my independence?* Although only 5% of people older than 65 live in nursing or residential facilities, roughly half the elderly population will eventually require assisted care by the end of life. And this is far more common for women after their spouses die first (Hinrichsen & Clougherty, 2006). A related fear: will my children and family members resent the burden of taking care of me?
>
> *When will I die and what happens afterward?* When you hit 60 and beyond, it is perfectly reasonable to wonder whether you will truly awake from a night's slumber or if you've been called by the specter of Death.

Even with the widespread prevalence of these fears and concerns, currently only 3% of older adults ever consult a mental health professional, and less than one-third of those experiencing major depression receive treatment (Hinrichsen &

Clougherty, 2006). As we are well aware, when an older patient does visit a physician, or is referred by family members, more often than not they are dismissed with prescriptions for antidepressant medication and sleeping pills.

JOYS OF WORKING WITH OLDER CLIENTS

Although we hear all kinds of enthusiastic comments from beginning therapists about how excited they are to work with children and adolescents, it is somewhat rare to hear a comparable level of enthusiasm for those who wish to specialize in helping the elderly. There are some obvious reasons for this—notably, there are (currently) more jobs available working with younger clientele and it also seems like it is far easier and more satisfying to offer help at a time in life when more serious problems might be prevented. Investing time in individuals who will enjoy a lifetime ahead of them to put the learning into practice may feel different than working with those who may only have a few years left to live. Nevertheless, there are not only certain advantages to working with older clients, but also some unique pleasures and satisfaction to working with this population (Fredman, Anderson, & Stott, 2010).

Working Systemically. It is interesting to work within a larger context of a client's world, which is virtually required when seeing older clients. This may include not only their immediate family and caregivers, but also their healthcare professionals and social support. This also allows us to find out what else is going on in the home, the efforts of other caregivers, and who else comes to visit or calls.

Working with Marginalized Groups

Older people have certainly been pushed to the edges of our culture, often experiencing discrimination, abuse, and neglect. Therapists who have a commitment to social justice and advocacy issues enjoy working with the elderly because they often don't have a voice to express their needs in a way they feel heard. Sometimes the elderly are almost shell-shocked when we ask them to sit down and tell us what is going on in their life.

"I'm interested in what you think about that and, especially, how you feel," a therapist remarked to an elderly client after he had talked about a recent incident that he found distressing. The man just kind of shrugged and gave a look that seemed to say, "Are you asking *me*? Are you sure you don't have me confused with someone else who has a life?"

Connecting to One's Own Family

Many therapists talk about how working with the elderly keeps them feeling connected to their own grandparents or parents who may have passed on. We all have memories of those significant elders who shaped our lives, whether a grandparent, teacher, or mentor. We look back with fondness and often feel regret for what we could have done to let them know how important they were to us. In some ways we are allowed to show our gratitude and respect by passing them forward to our older clients.

Listening to Wisdom. It is sometimes seen as a privilege to hear the stories and life lessons of those who have witnessed and experienced so much. These clients have such rich narratives about what they learned and experienced. Many talk about what they would do differently if they had a second chance to live life with their current insights.

Listening to a History Lesson

It is one thing to read about world events, or watch them in films, and quite another to hear from people who have actually lived during those turbulent times. The world changes rapidly throughout a lifetime and, without elders helping us to understand and appreciate these changes, we take too much for granted.

One of the aspects of our profession that is most interesting is the opportunity to learn so much about different facets of life. Every time we see a new client we learn about their profession and work, their loves and desires, and the best and worst parts of their life experiences. With older people there is so much more ground to cover, often about times in history that we've only read or heard about. What was it actually like to live through the Great Depression, the Korean War, the Civil Rights Movement, or Woodstock? Our older clients are walking (or sitting) history lessons.

Acquiring Inspiration

Therapists mention frequently how amazed they are by the resilience that some older people demonstrate, their determination to continue onward in the face of incredible obstacles and challenges. We feel inspired by their courage and, in some cases, the remarkable resilience they demonstrate dealing with struggles that seem unimaginably difficult.

JEFFREY: HISTORY LESSON

I was riding on a streetcar in Melbourne, Australia, when I caught an old man staring at me across the aisle. "Are you a Yank?" he yelled at me.

I cringed, thinking the crazy, old guy was mad at me for some reason. And I could barely understand him. "Excuse me?"

"A Yank? Are you from across The Pond?"

I wracked my brain, with no clue what he was talking about, until I realized he meant an American from the other side of the ocean. "Yes Sir," I finally mumbled.

"Ah ha! I thought so!" Then he leaned forward and started telling me that he had been only 15 years old when the Japanese were about to invade the city of Darwin in the Northern Territory. He immediately enlisted in the army and ended up fighting in the jungles of New Guinea in the most vicious hand-to-hand combat of World War II. "You Yanks saved us when the Poms were busy elsewhere."

He was talking about the Battle of Midway when the Australians realized that the Japanese fleet was headed their way. They begged the British for help but they were already overwhelmed dealing with the Nazis. It was the Americans who came to the rescue and stopped the Japanese cold in that critical naval battle. Without that intervention, the man explained to me that Australia would now be a part of Japan.

Although ordinarily I avoid such conversations in public places, especially with strangers, I was captivated by the old man's story. It taught me an important lesson—not only about a part of history, but also about the amazing life stories that are waiting to be heard if we are open to hearing them. I credit that conversation on the streetcar as the very beginning of my passionate interest in life narratives.

Creating Reciprocal Relationships

Therapists often report they enjoy a different kind of relationship with their older clients—one that is more informal in some ways, more porous in the usual boundaries, more personal and flexible.

Initiating Small Changes to Make a Big Difference

Sometimes it takes the littlest things to make a difference in the life of older people, and this is often reported as quite satisfying. Older clients are looking for changes in degree rather than a total change. Movement from something painful or toward something acceptable is what is sought. They are realistic about can possibly occur and yet serious about their involvement in the therapy process.

Appreciating the Importance of Life's Big Picture

It is important for the therapist to see adulthood as only one chapter in an older person's life. It can be so helpful and motivating to understand the complete picture of someone's life. We are a lot like books in that we are not composed of any one event or accomplishment, but are the product of many chapters instead.

Acknowledging Readiness to Change

Older clients are often uninterested in playing games and are in therapy for a specific, articulated purpose. With time running down, life is too short to spend it in a therapist's office unless there is something to be gained. This sense of urgency often makes older clients perfect candidates for what we do; they are also more inclined to follow through on what they say is important to accomplish. They may be less inclined to be defensive and more willing to accept feedback and to take responsibility for their actions. When older clients don't understand something, they will often be more likely to ask for clarification.

JON: NO TIME TO WASTE

I was teaching a wellness class to a large group of seniors at Elderhostel. At one point during the day I asked participants to divide into groups of six people and to choose group members they did not know very well. This task usually takes awhile to complete as people will mill around uncomfortably and lost. Inevitably, a few people will typically ask questions: "What do you mean by someone we don't know well?" "Is it okay if I join this group I work with even if we don't talk that much in the office?" "Can I take a break first and then join a group?" "You said a group of six people but this one has more than that." I must admit I held my breath because I anticipated it would take this group of seniors even longer to figure things out. To my surprise, however, it took them no more than 10 seconds for the groups to form. Before I could even regroup and plan what I wanted to say next, they were already yelling out to me, "Okay, we're ready! What do we do now?" It might have been my imagination but I swear they were already impatient because I was the one who was too slow for them.

Working with a Different Intent

Perhaps most important of all, therapists who work with elderly clients appreciate the increased flexibility and informality of the sessions. As people age, they tend to take things easier, loosen up, and, especially, enjoy interactions with those who are younger. They yearn for opportunities to share their stories and talk about their life experiences, especially without being continuously interrupted.

Talking about what he enjoys most when working with his many elderly clients, one therapist can't help but chuckle as he mentally sorts through a few in his caseload. "Twenty years ago, Frank was a CEO of a large corporation and now he is the volunteer greeter at a chiropractor's office, making sure everyone feels welcome and has coffee, tea, or water and a little bit of local gossip." The therapist shakes his head, recalling not only what a kick he gets out of listening to this man, but also how inspired he feels by him.

The therapist pauses for a moment, then signals he has another example. "Judy comes to see me two times each month and it seems to be the highlight of her month. Mine, too, in many ways. She always comes early and leaves late. She likes to hang out in my waiting room and talk with the secretary before our appointment. This is such a contrast with my own life because I'm always in such a hurry to get to the next task or the next place. She reminds me twice each month how I've got to learn to slow down. "Judy takes her time with everything she does, making every task a ritual. She makes herself a cup of tea just like it's part of some Japanese ceremony. For all I know, it is. My secretary and I always get a kick out of that after she leaves. Oh yeah, Judy also makes a point to bring us cookies she has baked for us—a special treat to share. She just wants to share her joyous bounty."

It is clear from these many examples that it is actually a special privilege to be able to work with older clients. They teach us things about their life, about the world, and even about ourselves and what is coming in the next chapter of our own lives.

CHAPTER 2

The Culture of Aging

The things I am supposed to be embarrassed about now—not being able to walk, not being able to wipe my ass, waking up some mornings wanting to cry—there is nothing innately embarrassing about them. It's the same for women not being thin enough, or men not being rich enough. It's just what our culture would have you believe. Don't believe it.

Mitch Albom, *Tuesdays with Morrie*

It's perhaps more than a little ironic that Ponce de Leon traveled to the New World in search of the Fountain of Youth. He eventually arrived in a place he called "Florida," which became a colony of elderly citizens (and he died of a poison arrow launched by an ungrateful inhabitant). The Spaniard was hardly the first to search for the eternal secret of youth. Alexander the Great spent considerable time, in between his conquests of the known world, also looking for this magical spring. And actually this search continues to this day; a culture of youth pervades almost every facet of daily life. Advertisements splashed across all media feature vibrant models of fresh, smiling faces atop youthful, vigorous bodies. People seek all kinds of magical elixirs to avoid the "ravages" of aging and present themselves to the world looking as young as possible, coloring hair, consulting surgeons, and purchasing all manner of potions, salves, creams, and vitamin supplements. We are living during a time when youth is celebrated universally over the experience of aging, and this despite the fact that close to 90% of all those older than 60 report feeling very confident and satisfied with their quality of life (National Council on Aging, 2013). Compare *that* with the feelings of most people in their 20s!

RECONFIGURED CONCEPTIONS OF OLD AGE

Throughout the study of human development, most major theorists virtually ignored anything that happened much beyond puberty. Likewise, any significant growth supposedly ceased during early adulthood, after which there was a long, slow slog toward infirmity. Jean Piaget's stages of cognitive development ended at formal operations during adolescence. Lawrence Kohlberg's stages of moral development pretty much stopped after formal schooling. Erik Erikson offered only two stages to cover everything that occurs after adolescence. Sigmund Freud (1905) had even less regard for potential learning and growth after childhood, believing that by the age of 50, "the elasticity of the mental processes on which treatment depends is, as a rule, lacking. Old people are no longer educable." Now the really interesting part of this statement is that Freud was in his 50s when he said this, suggesting that he was no longer qualified to participate in a process that requires tremendous "elasticity of mental processes." Yet, he went on complete his best work in the following two decades, producing some of his most creative ideas well into his 80s!

Until the 1960s, there was a myth perpetuated by psychologists and researchers that old age must necessarily be a time of disengagement. Unfortunately, many of these studies were based on observations and interviews with really sick and disabled elderly, not necessarily a representative normal population. In addition, although it does indeed appear that older people spend more time alone and are less inclined to be involved in a multitude of social activities, this isn't necessarily because they feel isolated, but rather because as people age they become far more selective and discriminating about how they spend their time. Although younger people might hang out with acquaintances or attend social gatherings rather than spend time alone, older people become more comfortable with solitude and make different choices to end superficial relationships or those they do not find satisfying (Cohen, 2005).

It has only been during the past few decades that the concept of aging has been completely reconfigured in such a way that it is not so much seen as a destiny of decrepitude and senility than as merely age-appropriate challenges that can be modified and adapted. Cohen (2006) mentions the year 1975 as a turning point in the ways our culture viewed the aging process. It was during that year that both the National Institute of Mental Health and the Veterans Administration launched ambitious research programs to study aging processes systematically, resulting in a transition away from viewing the process with a "problem focus" and instead looking at normal aging with minimal decline.

It was also Cohen's own research that brought increasing attention to the creative output still possible among elderly people. He cited one example in particular—folk art—in which the whole field is dominated by older artists who are making the most significant contributions. This is but one example of how cultural evolution has such a powerful influence on the ways that older people are viewed and treated, as well as how they see themselves. One very vibrant, passionate, and energetic older women talked openly about this struggle and the messages from others that she tries to deflect.

JON: MUSINGS OF AN OLDER THERAPIST IN THE CULTURE OF YOUTH

I am thrilled with the possibilities that my advanced age provides. Sure, I have learned to alter certain expectations, to slow down and pace myself differently. This has indeed been challenging, but of the greatest importance. I have been learning to respect my limits or else I pay for it later.

I enjoy living a far more thoughtful life. I have noticed a significant drop in my testosterone (my wife reports some relief!) and this has opened up new possibilities that I find refreshing. I had not realized just how much my life had been hormonally controlled. I also notice that people treat me differently, with more respect and reverence than before, perhaps because of my white hair and increasingly stooped gait.

I frequently remind myself how lucky I am just to be alive and in relatively good health. It was three years ago that I was supposed to die and now I am doing most of the things I did prior to the sickness, and I feel so fortunate that I chose a profession that allows me to work many years past traditional retirement age. And I also notice ways that I work differently now: my compassion and empathy and patience have deepened. I also recognize, and acknowledge, that in some ways I'm out of touch with the culture of youth and certainly not up to date with technology. My memory is a little slower but it performs with only a slight delay. Maybe I pause at remembering a name, book title, or date until the answer seems to magically appear a little later.

I have had to make a number of adjustments in my sessions, seeing fewer clients during a day, starting later in the morning and ending sooner. My sessions run longer than they used to. I also seem to enjoy what I'm doing more than ever.

"The most notable feeling about being 70 is the feeling of being a 'has-been.' Most younger people—sadly, including my kids—think that I don't really know much. And if I do, they know more. Our world has become so technologically dominated, and if you are not caught up in the latest tech, you are dismissed." She shakes her head in bewilderment at this current climate. "I feel that we've lost respect for ourselves and each other. Our culture has lost respect for the elders."

When she turned 70 this past year she was surprised by how hard it hit her viscerally. "Throughout the course of my life I have celebrated the decades, but this year I did not. I became lost and kind of sad. I started to remember, with great intensity, events in my life, the highs and lows, the stages of my education and my work life." She now feels immobilized and her work has come to a standstill. And it is those feelings of sadness and helplessness that led her to seek help. Yet, how many therapists are adequately prepared to address these issues and counteract the negative influences from our culture toward the elderly? Sadly, very few.

CULTURAL DIFFERENCES IN VIEWS OF AGING

Aging is less defined by biology than it is by cultural norms, beliefs, attitudes, traditions, and expectations (Cruikshank, 2009). Although in many Western locales the elderly are viewed as frail, dependent, lethargic, burdensome, and often marginalized and set out to pasture, other cultures revere elders as symbols of wisdom. People thus learn how to be old, just as they are taught how to view their elders. They also adopt the generalized attitudes and beliefs toward their position and status as an elder based on cultural conventions and "marketing" of messages. In America, for example, we spend more than $6 billion each year on miracle cures for aging—and that's a very conservative estimate (Gillick, 2006). This contributes to the "collective denial" of aging, masked by all the largely fraudulent potions and treatments that are supposedly designed to keep people looking young, including plastic surgery, Botox, hormone replacements, liposuction, potions, antioxidant creams, wrinkle removers, and snake oils.

There are strong cultural norms for what is considered "age appropriate" in every part of the world and in every era. Forms of entertainment throughout history often present the aged in particular ways, whether they were the plays of ancient Rome that portrayed older people as comic figures, or medieval literature in which overt hostility is expressed toward old men who take young lovers (Moody & Sasser, 2015). There are thus specific prescriptions in each culture for what is expected and considered acceptable in terms of dress, mannerisms, speech, and behavior. Nowhere is this more evident in our own culture in the ways that older men and women are held to very different standards. The stereotypical successful older man might be pictured in films (or on the street) as balding, portly, and climbing out of a convertible sports car accompanied by a young, leggy model. Compare that image with the stereotypical "little old gray-haired lady" hobbling along with a walker. Such cultural images, especially those perpetuated by the media, lead to all kinds of gross exaggerations and marginalization. And it is our job, in part, to counteract them by introducing and reinforcing alternative cultural scripts for what aging can mean.

Traditional models of the aging experience have been in direct conflict with one another during more recent times, either treating this stage of life in terms of "disengagement theory," a period of withdrawal and retirement from active life, as opposed to "activity theory," which postulates that it is useful and desirable to remain as productive and engaged as possible in the daily affairs of politics, family, work, and community.

"Age puzzles me," relates an older actress. "I thought it was a quiet time. My seventies were interesting and fairly serene, but my eighties are passionate. I grow more intense as I age" (Scott-Maswell, 1968, p. 6). Of course, which side we might align with would very much depend on the individual client's needs, interests, and ultimate goals, as well as their abilities and health.

An older therapist in his 70s relates how he frequently finds himself in conversation with friends who are a decade or two younger and ask what might lie ahead for them. "It's curious to me the range of reactions I hear from clients as well. Some say they can't wait to retire and kick back, let go of most of their current responsibilities, and others report they have no clue what they'd do and can never see themselves slowing down."

This particular therapist says that he so loves what he is doing that he can't wait to get started in the mornings. "I seem to have found wisdom, and with it some new ways to explain many things to clients and students that I never could before. It's as if I have hit another gear in my transmission that I didn't know even existed. I have never felt so on top of my game."

Older people are treated very differently in various work cultures. Some industries such as technology only seem to value youth, whereas others such as therapy value wisdom and experience. It is interesting how the status of the elderly has risen and declined throughout hunter–gatherer, agricultural, industrial, urbanization, and technological eras of human history. In the "modernization" theory of aging, it is surmised that status for the elderly changed as emphasis and needs of society also evolved, whether the emphasis was on land ownership, mobility, industrialization, or technology. As innovation and technology become more important, older people throughout history have often been devalued.

Among many indigenous cultures, the oldest citizens are treated with respect and status, and are afforded influential power within the tribe. The elders hold important judicial, political, and mentoring responsibilities. They are holders of tradition and history, storytellers who pass along cultural knowledge. In some groups they are empowered to select names for newborns, consulted on important decisions, or rule on disputes and mediate conflicts. They are considered sacred figures who enjoy closer relationships with God or the Spirit World. They lead community gatherings and bless the proceedings. Their permission and approval are sought for any major changes within the group.

Although older people in North America frequently report experiences of ageism, prejudice, and marginalization, this is not the case in many other cultures such as China, Singapore, and Trinidad, where people demonstrate much greater respect and reverence for the elderly (Tan, Zhang, & Fan, 2004). Other collectivistic cultures in the Middle East also provide much more support and caring within their families (Musaiger & D'Souza, 2009).

While tracing the cultural shifts in attitude toward older people, Freedman (1999) noted that a major change occurred during the 1820s in America, during the religious and social movements of the so-called Second Great Awakening. Elders were no longer treated with as much reverence and respect after this time. Seemingly within just a decade or two, the focus changed to an emphasis on novelty, youth, and progress, discarding anything—and anyone—associated with the old who "were portrayed as leftover relics from an outdated and regressive world—a past with little to teach the present" (Freedman, 1999, p. 43).

Lawrence-Lightfoot (2009) adds to this development by also mentioning how during the latter part of the 19th century older people became further infantilized and disrespected. No longer were distinguished men wearing powdered wigs or clothes with sloped shoulders to appear older; fashions changed to emphasize youth and vigor.

As Western cultures have become more industrialized and technologically dependent, ageism had become even more prevalent (Lee, 2009). Ancient, traditional wisdom is no longer considered a valuable resource for younger people when they can check Wikipedia or Google for anything they want to know. Certainly popular media has also had a huge impact, often portraying elderly people in negative ways as being helpless, dependent characters. Likewise, youth is celebrated in all kinds of ways as the model of desirability—and this value, perpetuated in the media and especially the advertising industry—influences young children's perceptions of the elderly at a very early age. In fact, the more television that people watch, the more likely they have negative views of older people (Donlon, Ashman, & Levy, 2005). They get the distinct impression that the elderly are either helpless victims or evildoers. Consider some of the classic older characters such as Mr. Scrooge, the Wicked Stepmother (*Cinderella*), Cruella de Vil (*101 Dalmatians*), the Mad Hatter (*Alice in Wonderland*), Rafiki (*The Lion King*), the witch from *Snow White*, and Grandpa from *The Simpsons*. It turns out that when older characters are portrayed in television, almost half the time they are featured in some stereotypically negative way as hapless, ineffectual, or downright evil. Such consistent portrayals in the media have an accumulative effect, even on older people themselves who are already struggling with issues of self-worth.

Individualism is now worshipped above all else, and anyone who doesn't demonstrate traits of fierce self-sufficiency is seen as a drain on the rest of us. Thus, rather than seeing older citizens as potential resources, beyond any grandparent responsibilities, they are usually discussed in the context of a burden, draining social security and taking up space.

SELF-PERCEPTIONS OF AGING INFLUENCED BY CULTURE

One of the prominent models of aging—socioemotional selectivity theory—postulates that aging is largely a cultural experience, shaped by the internalized values of the community (Carstensen, 2011; Fung, 2013). Furthermore, older people within a given culture are more amenable to adopting the dominant values and surrendering many of their previously articulated priorities. With time running down and the prospect of death an increasingly likely reality, it is suggested that taking on sanctioned norms more explicitly leads to its own kind of immortality because these beliefs will continue long after physical expiration. This means that older people are far more likely to accept the majority attitude toward the meaning of aging even when it conflicts with their personal worldview. No matter how productive, satisfied, and engaged they might feel toward their daily life, there will be overwhelming pressure to alter those self-perceptions to keep them in step with the party line.

Because cultural norms and social influences affect self-perceptions of aging almost as much as biological realities, it would seem that attitude is (almost) everything. Of course, this is an idea about which we are most familiar because most schools of psychotherapy include features that challenge "dominant narratives," "internalized scripts," "cognitive self-talk," "irrational beliefs," "colonized beliefs"—all of which refer to the ways people choose (or are pressured) to think about themselves in particular ways. This is no less true with the ways that people define who they are by their chronological age.

Marianne Corey, a prominent theoretician and textbook writer in the field, may be in her 70s but she doesn't see herself as necessarily old. "I have always been extremely active, physically very strong, and fiercely independent," she explained. Although she feels challenged to modify her activity level, and occasionally ask for help when she needs it, she feels it is important to be able to take care of herself. "I would much rather schlep my own suitcase than ask a porter to do it for me."

In her professional work, Marianne has to remind herself to adjust her schedule to compensate for increased fatigue. She mentions this, not as a limitation, but rather as a realistic acknowledgment of what she can handle. The challenge for her is not so much related to aging itself as it is to all the conflicting messages she hears from those around her about what she is supposed to be doing. Her husband, Jerry, who has not slowed down one iota, continues to pressure her to keep up to his pace. She gets other strong messages from her friends, children, and the larger culture that she should be settling down to her primary role as a grandmother. But, Marianne has always had a strong work ethic and feels it is important that she remain engaged professionally, at least to a certain extent.

One of the precious few developmental stages that covers later life, Erikson's concept of "generativity" is about the struggle to remain engaged with life and meaningful work rather than hitting a wall of stagnation. It refers to the concern for establishing and guiding the next generation, and is said to stem from a sense of optimism about humanity. It is through grandparenting, mentoring, teaching, and counseling others that people wish to leave their legacy in a number of different ways.

1. *A legacy of excellence*: This occurs when people strive to do their best every day, to increase their proficiency in a skill or add to their knowledge in some way. They serve as a role model for others, demonstrating a high standard

for learning and growth that never ends, and inspires others to follow a similar lead.

2. *A legacy of encouragement*: The traditional role for an elder in almost any culture was to support, mentor, and guide the younger generation. This is accomplished not just through sharing knowledge and wisdom, but also through encouragement. One new grandparent learned this lesson, discussing it in a session, when she discovered that all her attempts to "assist" her daughter-in-law with child-rearing advice were met with resistance and defensiveness. It didn't matter that the guidance was intended to be helpful and based on raising several children; it was perceived as critical and scolding. When this grandmother redefined her role as one of encouragement and support, it forged a different kind of relationship that made it safe for the mother to sometimes ask for help when and how she was ready to do so.
3. *A legacy of purpose*: People are most energized when they are using their strengths and talents for a purpose beyond themselves. To leave a legacy of purpose means that we care about something bigger than ourselves and our own self-interests. Although we are not going to live forever, our spirit and wisdom endures through the legacy we leave and the positive impact we make in our community.
4. *A legacy of love*: As each of us considers how and why we ended up in this profession, one common influence might be a family member or mentor who showed us compassion—and love—during times when we needed support the most. So much of what we do for others, beyond our therapeutic techniques and strategies, is to provide them with the caring for which they so desperately yearn.

Each of these legacies that are part of this stage of generativity are best described by George Bernard Shaw as a kind of mantra worth remembering, if not repeating. Shaw viewed himself in later life as belonging to his community as a whole, and felt a responsibility to work as hard and as long as he could to serve others. His life was no "brief candle," but rather a "sort of splendid torch which I have a hold of for the moment, and I want to make it burn as brightly as possible before handing it over to future generations."

CHALLENGING CULTURAL STEREOTYPES THAT ARE JUST PLAIN WRONG

There is a distinct image of older adults as lonely, isolated, depressed, discarded, living in the past, regretful, and embittered. This was certainly not the case with George Bernard Shaw, nor is it true for so many others who remain fully engaged with their lives and work more than ever as they age.

This first cultural stereotype that the elderly are lonely and isolated is clearly inaccurate. It is actually quite true that as we age our emotional responses do indeed change quite a bit, but in a different direction than has been generally assumed. In fact, there is considerable research demonstrating that older people are actually much more fulfilled than their younger counterparts (Leigland, Schulz, & Jankowsky, 2004; Riffin, Ong, & Bergman, 2014); they experience fewer negative emotions, and they are far more likely to feel satisfied. More often than not, they are at peace with themselves. One important reason for this is that although parts of the brain will inevitably lose volume and functionality with aging the amygdala (which controls emotional responses) becomes much less active. This is one reason why older people don't become nearly as upset about little things that might bother others who are younger.

Even more surprising is recent research challenging the idea that brain cells die with age and are never rejuvenated. It turns out that new neurons are constantly being reformed throughout the life span, and their rate of restoration is directly related to the degree of cognitive activity that still takes place. This leads to the support of one stereotype: use your brain actively or lose it. New advances in cognitive training, combined with physical exercise, lead to increased neuroplasticity (Zolyniak, Schulte-Gocking, & Kraft, 2014).

This has profound implications for ways we might reconceptualize the role of psychotherapy for older people in that one of our jobs may involve brain stimulation—that is, facilitating conversations that trigger mental exercise and stretch cognitive processing with challenging ideas. We could very well use some of the strategies of speech therapists and occupational therapists that assist in the rehabilitation of stroke survivors in much the same way personal trainers support and encourage more vigorous workouts. This expands our conversations with older clients not only to talk about problems and challenges, but also to strengthen their cognitive functioning by exercising the mind, whether through crossword puzzles, Scrabble, card games, daily meditation, or brain teasers.

Our redefined roles with aging clients could focus less on resolving conflicts and fixing problems—many of which are not amenable to change—and also to stimulate and energize thinking in creative ways, as well as help them to exercise their brain in a variety of constructive ways. For this to work most smoothly, it would first be important to help them to challenge many of the limiting beliefs and attitudes that get in the way, many of which are the result of biased and inaccurate cultural scripts. Like people of any age, older indvidiuals become what they think about themselves. This may also compromise their recovery from disabilities as well as open up new opportunities for growth and learning (Levy, Slade, Murphy, & Gill, 2012). Examples of such internalized beliefs include the following:

- "I'm disabled and too crippled ever to regain adequate functioning."
- "I'm too old to change."
- "I forget things and there's nothing I can do about it."

- "I might as well accept my situation since I'm over the hill anyway."
- "Nobody cares about an old fogey like me."
- "Therapy can't help someone as old as me."
- "You can't teach an old dog new tricks."

None of these statements are necessarily accurate and all are amenable to being questioned, if not challenged vigorously. A man in his 70s in the last stages of prostate cancer was feeling especially discouraged and despondent about the ways his sex life had changed as a result of "medical castration" to lower testosterone levels (designed to increase longevity). "My notions of love, caring, energy, and physical sex all changed so dramatically, practically overnight. When I was young, so much of my life was ruled by the need for physical sex, then the sexual desire slowly diminished to the point that I became incredibly frustrated."

He had been told by doctors, and influenced by culture, that as an older man his sex life would have been pretty much over anyway, so it wasn't that much of a loss. But, he refused to accept this sentence and that he had to abandon his identity as a sexual being.

"I had to learn to be open and laugh at the these changes and frustrations, and enjoy a new kind of intimacy." It helped that his wife was so supportive and understanding (although she was dealing with her own changes), aiding his adjustment to a different way of understanding sexual intimacy. "Although our sexual encounters became less frequent, I learned the importance of physical contact. Simple things like being physically close, holding hands, and verbally expressing our love became more and more significant and, honestly, plain wonderful. The constant desire and perceived need for intercourse has become a welcome loss, and our loving so much softer and calm."

SPECIAL CULTURAL CHALLENGES FOR AGING WOMEN

As different as men and women are in so many ways, the distinctions can become even more pronounced with age. Physical attractiveness has always been the currency, the gold standard, for women's self-image and value by others. When their hair goes gray; wrinkles, sags, and age spots appear; and their waistline bulges, women may often experience a loss of value, vitality, power, and self-worth (Crose, 2002).

When looking at the culture of aging, it is not surprising that women would end up with some special challenges. Not only are women held to a different standard of what it means to be old, but as a function of higher life expectancy, also face many of these difficulties alone. The average woman faces about 14 years of life as widows (at least for those married to men) compared with half that time for men.

When men become older, turn gray or lose their hair altogether, and develop a paunch and wrinkles, they are considered "distinguished," but for many women such signs of aging supposedly lessen their value. So much of the cosmetics and plastic surgery industries are focused on selling anti-aging solutions to women, coloring hair, installing implants or collagen, and offering an assortment of makeup, creams, and other products to disguise, if not fend off, the most overt signs of aging. An older man who loses a spouse will find it far easier to find a new, younger replacement whereas a woman in that predicament will have far fewer options.

Although elderly men might be described as "geezers" (that is, tottering old fools), women are subjected to even more cruel stereotypes—"the little old lady, perhaps with tennis shoes, unfashionably dressed, unstylish grey hair, and unadorned with either makeup up or jewelry" (Gergen, 2009, p. 253). Another version of negative stereotype would be "battle-ax"—the overbearing, aggressive, domineering woman who is a perceived threat to the dominance of men. Or the "crone," the old witch, who is demanding and manipulative.

Beginning at the relatively early age of 50, women are labeled as "menopausal," which is subtext for emotionally unstable. After the childbearing years are over, women were traditionally viewed as having little value, which is not surprising considering the ways that youth and masculinity have been venerated. Within our own field, Freud's (1927) own negative biases set a precedent, describing most women as passive, opposed to change, and with little initiative or much to contribute. Even his own daughter and designated champion was encouraged only to guard her father's ideas zealously, rather than contribute anything creative or novel on her own.

As a function of outliving men, women are also far more likely to suffer extended losses and deal with grief issues. It is not only probable they will outlive a male partner, but also they will struggle with bereavement issues related to increased social isolation. Feminist approaches to working with older women explore the underlying (or overt) sense of worthlessness by helping them to reconnect with their roles as heroic elders who play an important role mentoring the next generation.

Shirley, age 71, talks in therapy about how her entire life has been devoted to her appearance. She still feels the same internal pressure to look her best although it feels like nobody even notices her anymore. "It is as if I disappeared in my late 40s, which is so strange considering that when I was younger it seemed like people gawked at my beauty. I was what they called a 'looker' or a 'major babe.' "

Shirley shakes her head in bewilderment and wonders where that person vanished and when that change happened. Then, she looks up with a sad smile. "Now

I remember. It was on my 49th birthday. One day I was young and gorgeous and then I was gone, invisible, no more."

Shirley insists that, in truth, she doesn't really mind aging at all, but the transition to thinking of herself as old, and being treated that way, is taking some time to adjust. "Now I am enjoying being something more than just a pretty face. I was forced to realize that I have some real talents. I have a brain, a personality, a sense of humor, and all the things that I didn't even know existed. I am no longer just a sex object."

Shirley notices that her husband has gone through a parallel process of adaptation. "All he used to think about was sex. But, as his urges diminish, he seems to see me more for who I am in a multitude of ways he missed earlier. I don't look so gorgeous and he doesn't seem to care so much. We have learned to appreciate other more important things in ourselves."

Therapy can assist older people in so many ways with these issues, as illustrated in one more example. Nadya's husband died of cancer more than 20 years ago. Until that time she had been a dutiful wife who fulfilled her expected roles as dictated by her culture and family. While her husband worked as an engineer for an automotive company, she took care of the home and children, and supported him in all the ways he needed. She had been more than happy to follow his lead with respect to their interests and social activities, rarely traveling except to football games at the university they had both attended. Their interactions revolved mostly around their children, their religious activities, and the annual trip they would take with alumni from the university. Otherwise, they lived a mostly quiet, ordinary, and satisfying life.

When Nadya's husband died, she was, at first, bereft. She had never had to make decisions on her own or, in fact, decide much of anything because her husband had always made such arrangements. She had never even considered what she wanted to do because she had been content to follow her husband's lead. Fortunately, her loyalty (and fiscal management) was rewarded with sufficient funds that she would not have to worry much about finances.

After a period of mourning and adjustment, Nadya decided, at age 70, that it was time to reinvent herself. She became an inveterate traveler. Although previously she had not ventured beyond cities that held an annual bowl game where their alma mater played, Nadya now wanted to see the world—and she did so with passion and dedication.

One approach that is focused specifically on addressing some of the cultural scripts related to what it means to be an aging woman borrows from the "motherline archetype" (Trotman & Brody, 2002). When older women feel isolated, discarded, and estranged, even worthless, it is useful to help them to connect again with their mothers and grandmothers, and, if appropriate, their own maternal roles in life. For older female therapists, this task is even more important because of the ways they can serve as role models for their female clients.

Aging can provide some real breakthroughs that allow some women like Shirley and Nadya to make amazing life changes. There are many women who have lived longer than their predecessors who are carving out satisfying lives. And there are many women elders, many of them psychotherapists, who serve as role models for all their clients about how people can indeed age proudly and gracefully no matter what messages still echo throughout the dominant culture.

THE CULTURES OF GENERATIONAL COHORTS

Although we have discussed at length how cultural values within the community influence and impact the aging process, as well as how older people view their worth, there are also implicit and dominant attitudes within the therapy profession that have compromised the care of older clients, or at least their access to services. We are all about facilitating change, the more and faster the better.

Ask a therapist, almost any therapist, to describe an ideal client and the answer hasn't changed that much since the early research on YAVIS preferences—clients who are young, attractive, verbal, intelligent, and successful. Very few would honestly say they prefer working with clients who present chronic, intractable conditions; tend to ramble and lose focus; have compromised cognitive functioning; and have no meaningful job. But of course, this is hardly the case with the vast majority of older people, regardless of the perceptions.

JEFFREY: THE CLUELESSNESS OF A YOUNG THERAPIST

When I was a young man I volunteered to lead a therapy group at a residential community for older people. Groups were my expertise and I had worked with all kinds of populations and settings, so I surely felt the confidence to deal with this situation.

By the time I arrived in the room there were about 20 of the residents waiting for me, 19 women and one man who I noticed was being attended to by several of those seated next to him. He had a grin on his face as if this was his harem.

It took some time—okay, it took a very long time—to rearrange the chairs into a circle. A few of the participants insisted they couldn't hear my "lecture" if they were sitting too far away. Others insisted that they always sat in the same place and didn't feel comfortable relocating to another space.

After explaining that I wouldn't be talking to them but rather helping them to tell their own stories, a few of the people raised their hands to ask me questions about my age, whether I was married, and how many children I had, and one of the women told me I was way too young to be a doctor. I smiled and gritted my teeth.

"So," I got us started, "who would like to begin by saying something about what you'd like to talk about today?"

One woman immediately raised her hand and I heard others groan and saw eyes rolling. "Well young man," she said in a shrill voice, "I'm glad you asked."

That was it. That was essentially the end of the group. The woman spoke nonstop for 20 minutes and there was absolutely nothing I could do to stop or even interrupt her. She was on a roll and obviously had a lot she wanted to say about all kinds of things. I was fascinated by the way she could seemingly speak without stopping for a breath. There were others who tried to get a word in but she would hold up an arthritic hand and give them the death stare until they backed down. When I tried to offer a supportive comment or reflect one tiny part of her monologue that continued at such a speed I could barely hold on to a piece, she would give me that withering stare to back me down. I was terrified of her.

I could see others shaking their heads in frustration, although they were apparently used to this behavior. So, they began ignoring her altogether and engaging in their own conversations with those near them, although one woman was yelling across the room at her friend who couldn't hear what she was asking. I was fascinated because the one guy in the room was enjoying a neck massage from one of the women sitting next to him. He was the only one in the room who seemed oblivious to whatever was going on, just enjoying the personal attention.

Everyone politely thanked me after the group ended, with nobody else really having the chance to say much. The one women who did all the talking just scowled at me and repeated the comment that I was too young to be a doctor. And that ended my first experience doing "therapy" with older adults. I was 26 years old.

Much has been made in our field about the critical importance of sensitivity to cultural diversity issues. Many conference proposals, as well as book and article submissions, are virtually required to address multicultural issues before they are considered sufficiently relevant and appropriate for dissemination to the profession. Courses in diversity are required in graduate school and continuing education credits. And almost all the attention is directed to diversity with respect to ethnicity, race, religion, socioeconomic status, gender, and sexual orientation. Yet, age cohorts are just as much a cultural phenomenon as any other characteristic we might consider.

"The Greatest Generation" was born during the first two decades of the 20th century and are defined, in part, by surviving the years through the Great Depression and the Second World War. "The Silent Generation" included children during the Second World War and, to some extent, have been characterized by their work ethic. Then came the "Baby Boomers," who are currently dominating the aging population, most of them coming of age during the turbulent '60s with the Vietnam War. Their children are often referred to as "Millennials" or the "MTV Generation," growing up during the spectacular growth of technology and the Internet. "Gen X" and "Gen Y" are now following as the next generational cohorts, each marked by their own history, customs, media and social preferences, and distinct values.

Given that the older cohort that is now most prevalent (or about to be) among our aging clients consists of Baby Boomers, younger therapists will be required to develop cultural sensitivity and awareness of the music, seminal television shows and films, as well as fluency in the language usages of this group. For instance, a number of common expressions of people currently in their 70s and 80s use terms that are now endangered, if not totally extinct.

- *"You sound like a broken record."* Records were round disks that played music on a device called a *turntable.*
- *"That's a Kodak moment."* Kodak was a company that made something called *film* to record photographs.
- *"That's nothing to write home about."* In the prior century people used to write family members on paper—with a pen! They'd put the message in an envelope and actually pay money for a stamp. It would actually take several days to arrive at its destination.
- *"He was asleep at the switch."* This is an old railroad term—before automation—that refers to a worker who was bored.
- *"Dial her up."* Telephones, actual landlines, had to be turned in a circular rotation for each number before push-button phones came on the scene.

We mention these as examples of the cultural uniqueness of each generational cohort and how, just as we would need to educate ourselves about any other diverse group, such as Seventh Day Adventists, Bangladeshi Americans, undocumented immigrants, or the homeless, we need to become aware of the unique experiences that helped to shape older people and their values. Of course, the diversity among any generational cohort, based on their religion, ethnicity, race, geographic location, and other factors, is just as great as what we have learned to appreciate throughout any other period of the life span. If anything, such differences might be more pronounced because of significant advances in social movements that address racism and economic disparity, gender bias, homophobia, and religious intolerance during the past several decades.

This chapter has explored what it means to be "age appropriate" in the context of cultural scripts that often limit the ways older people see themselves, as well as how they are seen by others. As never before in the history of the human race, being old is taking on new meaning and offering new and different opportunities. Our job, as therapists, is to help our older clients challenge many of their assumptions and perceptions that compromise their desire to become more engaged with active life.

PART II

The Aging Therapist

CHAPTER 3
The Senior Therapist

Growing old is not for sissies.
Bette Davis

As any physicist will tell you, it is the nature of things to fall apart. This is called *entropy,* the second law of thermodynamics that refers to the inevitable wear and tear on machines—and living things—that take their toll over time. All things eventually break down, and this is perhaps the most pervasive phenomenon in Nature. The sun will burn itself out like a light bulb. Earth is slowing down on its axis. Ice will melt. Nations collapse. Order will turn into disorder. And every therapist, no matter how brilliant and accomplished, will eventually lose some of the faculties that were once relied on to produce successful outcomes. Memory will become less precise. Fatigue will replace boundless energy. And a once laserlike mind will become less focused even as it continues to burn brightly. Adaptations and adjustments are not only desirable but absolutely necessary if the senior therapist is to maintain consistent levels of productivity and excellence.

THE MATURATION OF INTUITION

Senior status as a therapist is supposed to be a time of reverence and prestige, and indeed it does come with certain privileges that are not afforded to beginners in the field. But it is also a kind of adolescence all over again, a time of extreme adjustments to changes in the body, changes in societal expectations, but with a lot more baggage. Questions are asked: "Is this the best I'm ever going to feel?" "Is the best I'm ever going to do?" "Is this as good as it gets?"

With age you can actually measure growth and deterioration at various life stages. Although once upon a time you could run a seven-minute mile, sleep through the night without waking, remember almost everything in a session, or see 10 clients a day without much difficulty, aging brings new challenges—and new gifts.

Perhaps one of the biggest changes is that senior therapists trust their intuition. One way to think about the intuitive process is that it essentially represents an immediate and deep understanding of underlying patterns based on experience. It often bypasses conscious or even rational thought, relying on a kind of instant feeling about what might be going on. Yalom (2015) is sometimes intrigued by the ways he has matured as a therapist in old age, willing to take risks that he would not have been inclined to do earlier in his career: "I've grown to trust my unconscious to behave in a professionally responsible manner, and I know full well that it is not so much *what* I say about my thoughts that is important but rather *that I am willing to express them*" (p. 22).

What may appear as stabs in the dark to the uninitiated are actually examples of pattern recognition that have been formed and catalogued throughout decades of practice. "Sometimes it seems like I've heard and seen it all before," one senior therapist admits. "Or maybe it's just that I seem to be able to react so quickly to situations that would take so much longer when I was younger. I notice things in voice tone and inflection that would have escaped me previously. Oh, there are things I miss as well, things I might have picked up on when I encountered something for the first time. I miss some little things, forget some details, but I can get to the essence of an issue with a depth, an intensity, and a swiftness that still surprises me."

CHALLENGING THE USUAL RULES

For reasons unclear to us, there has been a certain reluctance to discuss the subject of aging as it applies to therapists, and actually very little has been written about this subject. It is also not an issue that comes up very often at conferences, although it is likely one of the most pressing concerns on the minds of half our guild. One therapist, who just turned 65, admitted he was less than eager to talk about his feelings because of his changing identity in the way he saw himself and the ways he was now viewed by others.

"I was at a conference recently," he mentioned as an example, "and I looked around the room a couple of times and saw all these young, enthusiastic faces and I thought to myself, 'I used to be like that, too.' It just made me feel even older."

It isn't just that he feels older, but also that he notices that he operates quite differently in session than he used to. He still holds a very optimistic view of clients' ability to change, but he also finds he is more realistic about what can actually be accomplished, as well as the limits of what is possible.

This deep understanding flies in the face of many of the new breed of younger therapists who are applying chemical and brain solutions to what the senior therapists just seem to know and understand. It may appear as if the younger professionals are objectifying and making a science out of what is an art form for many of the senior therapists. Many older therapists developed their knowledge and understanding through experience and trial and error, whereas many of today's clinicians are more grounded in research and empirically validated treatments. They are conceptualizing treatment much more like a medical professional trying to remove symptoms rather than repairing deep wounds that are the result of neglect, dysfunction, and lack of attachment.

A number of years ago, Tallmer (1992) interviewed and surveyed more than 100 older psychoanalysts, as well as elders in the profession who represent other orientations (Carl Rogers, John Bowlby, Robert Havighurst, and B. F. Skinner). She was particularly interested in the ways they have changed and adapted in their work as they have gotten older. Most of the participants in the study reported they had become more flexible, outspoken, and free from "rules" they found oppressive and irrelevant to the needs of their clients.

As just one example of this, we remember interviewing Arnold Lazarus, (Kottler & Carlson, 2003) noted cognitive and multimodal theorist, who described a case in which a man found it difficult to engage in any kind of relationship with women; he was terrified of approaching them and had extremely poor social skills. Lazarus found it a little ridiculous just to sit around and talk about this skill deficit and, instead, invited the man to join him at a bar, where he proceeded to support, encourage, and coach the client to approach various women and then process the rejections afterward. More and more often, Lazarus had found that certain boundaries were designed more to protect therapists than actually to help clients in ways they needed assistance the most.

In Tallmer's survey and interviews, the older therapists also reported they were less inclined to pathologize behavior, redefining "normality" far more broadly. Similarly, they were less inclined to judge themselves or others in more absolute terms, instead feeling as if they were more realistic and modest in their expectations for themselves and their clients. Because most of them were psychodynamic in approach, they also mentioned that transference phenomena were much easier to navigate as a result of their appearance as grandparent figures and less as erotic objects. In addition, they felt they were much more honest and accurate in assessing their own capabilities. One 83-year-old therapist, for example, talked about the adjustments she made in the latter years, particularly with regard to reduced energy and vitality: "At such times I reduced demands on myself, and after a few weeks felt ready to be intensely involved again" (Tallmer, 1992, p. 394).

One area that was problematic for many of the senior therapists is that they had lost a number of clients and were receiving significantly fewer referrals from colleagues. Yet they were reluctant to reach out to those sources, or ask colleagues for help, because they felt some shame at their loss of stature or reduced demand. They didn't see this as much as age discrimination as the inevitable result of being less visible, although some reported frustration that certain jobs were no longer open to them.

SENIOR STATUS AND THE ART OF PSYCHOTHERAPY

The persona of an aging therapist, especially an elderly, male psychoanalyst, presents an image that is quite different from a younger version today that is far more likely to be female and a person of color. There is also little doubt that a distinctive aura is created by the distinguished elder, one that triggers all kinds of reactions in clients, both positive and negative. Certainly there is less to prove, perhaps less narcissism and fear of failure, but also an increased sense of impoverishment in other areas of life that may make professional work and relationships with clients even more important (Chessick, 2013).

Michael Hoyt, a noted Ericksonian and brief therapist, has witnessed many of the major changes in the field during his 40 years of practice, mostly for a large health organization. "I've increasingly experienced the unrelenting pressure for more productivity—"More intakes! More groups!"—and more documentation," he said with exasperation. "Being older [bald pate with fringe of white hair and goatee], clients often relate to me now in a more avuncular/grandfatherly way than when I was younger. Sometimes this gives an advantageous aura of experience and wisdom, but sometimes it also suggests, not always incorrectly, of being unaware of recent styles and trends." It boggles his mind sometimes that when he was in his 30s he used to counsel older people about later life issues. "Now I'm aware of a cultural gap talking to 20-somethings: '*Habla usted*?' 'Hook-up?' 'Selfie?' 'Four-thousand-dollar apartments?' "

In truth, Hoyt has worked much harder than most to stay current on contemporary trends and cultural knowledge. Although he has been transitioning into semiretirement, he still hungers for new challenges. A lifetime of experience has taught him that, although his repertoire and style will essentially remain intact, he has gotten so much better at "discerning which clients I can help and which ones don't match so well with what I do best."

This awareness of his limits and strengths is absolutely crucial. considering the very real challenges he faces in continuing to remain professionally active. He notices that sometimes it's hard to "stay on" in sessions—to remain sharp, attentive, and creative. Nevertheless, he uses other ways of compensating for these changes. "I remember reading that as Willie Mays [baseball legend] aged, he may not have been quite so quick afoot, but he made up for it by knowing more about what was likely to happen, and so where and how to make adjustments with his batting stance or position in the outfield."

Hoyt also recognizes there is something special about the "beginner's mind"—that fresh innocence and enthusiasm and unbridled passion that can be so contagious. "I try to strike a balance between the wisdom of experience—seeing where things are likely to go and what might be most helpful—with the freshness of someone who is just starting out in the field. This means seeing each person and moment as unique, rather than just another case of codependency or marital conflict or anxiety."

What Hoyt especially appreciates about this stage of his career is that, although there is increased pressure from health maintenance organizations to engage in superficial symptom reduction, he still finds ways to help people—and himself in a parallel process—to "discover more meaning and satisfaction in life at a time when I feel so much more interest in such existential issues." This highlights another facet of what it means to be a senior therapist—the increased flexibility and pragmatism. During our interviews with the greatest living (and elderly) theoreticians of the past era, including Jay Haley, William Glasser, Albert Ellis, Virginia Satir, Arnold Lazarus, Peggy Papp, Nick Cummings, John Krumboltz, Lenore Walker, and so many others, we have found consistently that, although they might be known for developing a particular model, they have actually become much more willing to borrow ideas from so many other approaches, much more integrative as they aged.

"Theories come and go," Hoyt observed. "But what it all comes down to is a positive alliance, honesty, compassion, and courage. That's what matters the most. The research data seem to say that we're not getting better outcomes than we used to. People are resilient—except for those who aren't." He mentions this as just one example of a central thesis he enjoys teaching to younger colleagues he supervises and mentors. And that leads to one of the most important roles of all for a senior therapist: the opportunity and responsibility to serve as a model for the next generation of practitioners.

After conducting well more than 50,000 therapy sessions during his long and distinguished career, Hoyt reflects on how it has impacted him. "I may not have heard it all, but I've heard a lot. I'm seldom shocked by anything I encounter. I've seen from my patients what works and what doesn't, and learned from them how to cope more gracefully with things in my own life. I still have curiosity, hope, love, and compassion, but also greater awareness of the finitude of life. This has helped me to spend more of my time doing other, nontherapy things rather than spending all day in the office listening to people—especially listening to their miseries."

In some ways, Hoyt is also less patient with endless complaining that doesn't lead anywhere constructive. With less time left in his life, and with friends and colleagues falling apart, he feels a heightened urgency to get things done. "I've also found myself, at times, being envious as I sit in my office listening to adventures my clients are out having. Am I going to spend my whole life in this room?" Meanwhile, his biological clock keeps ticking along, motivating him to become more engaged in the things that matter most.

AGING ALONGSIDE OUR CLIENTS

Senior therapists come in all different shapes, sizes, theoretical orientations, and ages. Hedda Bolgar was interviewed as perhaps the oldest living therapist still in active practice (Lopez, 2011). At age 103 she was still seeing clients four days per week in addition to her lecture and supervision commitments, with no immediate plans to cut back her workload. Even after all those years, she still remained fascinated by the conversations that take place in sessions, still intrigued by the ways that people have the capacity to reinvent themselves. Although she has had more than her share of adversity; and lived through wars, famines, and the death of her spouse; she remained energized and passionate about continuing to help those who trust her. She felt she was put on this earth to make a difference and accomplish certain things. "I'm so far behind I can never die," she says laughing.

Talking about the changes that have taken place in her work as she has aged during 40 years of practice, Saralie Pennington (2009) also reflected on the parallel process she has witnessed in both her clients and her own development over time. She asked her long-term clients, those she had been seeing for many years or even decades, about what they observed was different now than previously. With good humor she said, "One client said she thought I was a little more forgetful about times and dates, but then again it might be her own faulty memory because she too was aging, and that yes she noticed my face had changed but that she liked how it was changing" (p. 207).

Consistent with her feminist leanings, Pennington considers it a privilege to be able to age alongside her clients, an opportunity for a kind of shared positive redefinition of what it means to be an older woman. That is one aspect of the field that she has always found so fulfilling—that it isn't just about healing wounds, but about creative growth as part of the aging process.

THE THERAPIST'S OWN AGING

In one sense aging comes as an epiphany. We have always been told that human development is gradual, incremental, and virtually unnoticeable because of its glacial progression, but it sometimes seems that growing old occurs as one swift, jarring realization. Until about age 60, Virginia Lawson Clower (1992) observed, while looking in the mirror, that she felt she was essentially unchanged. A little gray hair here and there. Bifocals. A few bulges and a bit of weight gain. But otherwise not much felt all that different from her youth. Then it seemed that denial was no longer possible: the effects could not be ignored once illnesses struck—and she realized, upon recovery, that she'd never be as good as new again. It is one thing to come to terms with one's own loss of mobility and mental acuity but quite another to navigate these issues with clients. Clower sees clearly how clients pretend to ignore her memory lapses, or her involuntary gasps from some ache or pain, but there's little doubt there is a difference in how she works in sessions. If nothing else, she thinks about death a lot more, always lurking in the background. And there are all the inconveniences and annoyances of everything taking a little longer and a lot slower. It is only by growing old herself that she can finally appreciate the sort of everyday problems her older clients talk about in sessions that may once have just seemed like endless whining and complaining.

Although Clower was in good health, with no major disabilities, she was *different* than she'd ever been before. And although many of these changes were losses—of vitality and clarity—there were also some significant gains, especially a curiosity about things she never noticed before. She has learned to reach out to others more than ever before, to ask for help when she needs it. After 40 years of practice, she admitted she was tired and had to slow down the pace of her work and restructure the way she worked. She reinvented herself in later life and redefined her identity as a therapist, respecting the limits of what was feasible and comfortable for her. She remembered that Anna Freud observed that treating an adolescent was similar to running next to a train. And that is also how coming to terms with aging felt to her, trying to catch up to something that is always out of reach.

In the same collection of essays about how elderly psychiatrists experience aging, Eckardt (1992) does not feel the "hard edge" of decline much at all. At 76, she admits to living the same "agreeable rhythms of life" that have been familiar during later adulthood. She admits to an awareness of bodily changes but not to the extent that she feels all that limited. She talked to her age mates about their own views on the subject and their responses seemed consistently that it's best not to think about the future very much. The view of the future for the elderly "is shaped by the certainty of death, certainty of physical decline, and a total unpredictability of the character and quality of our final years" (p. 87).

Eckardt realizes that if the future seems depressing to some among elderly therapists, and others, it is because they have dreams and aspirations that have been unfulfilled. Although it is certainly true that all of us have some ideas that we've never followed through, or ambitions we never realized, Eckardt doesn't see old age as the end, but rather a kind of new beginning. It is a time for reassessment and adjustment.

So-called "retirement," whether partial or complete, is essentially about freeing time to do things never possible earlier in life. For therapists who have remained vital and active and completely engaged all their lives, this developmental task presents some special challenges, but nobody else is better equipped to deal with it. What we've done for a living is help people to face the realities of what is possible, and what is not, and to proceed accordingly. As such, the infirmities and limitations of age can be viewed as mild annoyances, not as major impediments to deeper (and different) engagement with life. According to Eckardt (1992), this stage of life provides a number of opportunities to let go of some responsibilities and obligations, replacing them with new and thrilling adventures. Eckardt seems to capture our excitement with the many possibilities that face our future time on this planet.

When she was a few years younger, Eckardt worked with an elderly client who was, in some ways, her teacher about what it meant to grow old. What brought the woman to therapy in the first place was her interest in exploring what to do with the time she had left. The woman admitted she had enjoyed a rich life, filled with travel to exotic places, a meaningful career, and a lovely family, but she had always been someone's wife or daughter or grandmother. "Now it is time to learn," she announced. "Now it is time for adventure. Now it is time for truth. Now it is time for me" (Eckardt, 1992, p. 93). The sessions that unfolded thereafter were related to helping this woman find her voice, without as much concern for how others might react. However, it has been our experience that so many of the people who reach this place and find themselves are most concerned with social interests and how they can help others.

There's the joke about the elderly guy who was being interviewed for a job by the director of human resources. "What would you say is your greatest weakness?" the manager asked the fellow.

"I'd say honesty," the applicant immediately answered.

"Well," the manager paused, "I wouldn't say that honesty is exactly a weakness."

"You know," the older man replied, "I don't really give a shit what you think." There is indeed a certain freedom in not caring so much about cultural restraints that sometimes have been more debilitating than any physical decline.

LEARNING TO ADAPT TO AGING

Jerry Corey, one of the premier and influential textbook authors in the field, believed that very little has changed for him as a therapist and supervisor as he reached 80 years of age. He still feels as much passion and enthusiasm for his work as when he began a half century ago. "Mentoring has been a passion of mine since I began teaching in the early 1960s," he revealed. "I feel a sense of accomplishment when younger therapists I've worked with come back years later and let me know how they dared to dream the impossible dream, and how they exceeded goals and visions they had for themselves."

Corey is quick to point out to them that, although he didn't do this for them, he does accept responsibility for encouraging and challenging them to find their hidden talents. He feels so proud of the things they are now doing in their lives and feels honored that he was a small part of their success that now has so many significant ripple effects on others they are now helping.

Corey also is a little surprised by the extent to which he still manages to remain completely engaged in the lives of those he is helping. "I never tire of hearing client stories or feel the least jaded by the suffering of people in my groups. Every story is new and fresh, and I still feel touched by them."

That's not to say that he doesn't feel challenged in some ways now that he is older. "I have to continue to remind myself that I am only one person and can do only so much. I am very slowly realizing that I take on too much at times and have difficulty saying no." This is often a common theme among aging professionals—that is, realizing the limits of what we are capable of doing.

Corey has gotten better at turning down invitations now that he has more trouble with the discomforts and annoyances of travel. He receives many invitations to present at conferences or deliver keynote speeches around the world, but he finds it exhausting and disorienting to adjust to the different time zones and locations. Lately he's been saying no a lot more than yes to such opportunities. "I am not flexible when it comes to adjusting to the demands of travel and working abroad, and as I age I'm getting even more rigid and set in my ways."

He also noticed that with respect to his writing, it takes him a lot longer to produce a chapter. There are several reasons for this, most obviously the awareness that it takes him longer to do anything as an older person, but new technology also has an inhibiting effect, making it harder for him to adjust to different ways of doing things. "I find much of the new stuff to be incredibly frustrating to learn and I seem to be a slow learner. I often wish I could have stayed with my yellow pad and pen."

Although he's reluctant to admit it, Corey acknowledges that he's also experienced some physical challenges. "My five year old granddaughter tells me all the time, 'Papa, you should go to a hearing doctor.' Yeah, I've been slow to admit that this is a problem for me and I typically blame others for not talking loud enough."

Corey also discloses his memory is failing—that he will go into a room to get something and then forget why he is there. His 94-year-old mother was a role model for him. He remembers that whenever she would forget something or get lost in the middle of a sentence, she'd just shrug unconcernedly and say that it would come back to her if she just waited awhile. "She showed me how to accept these little annoyances and frustrations rather than being overcome by them."

It's interesting the way he had a model for successful adaptation to aging that is now so helpful to him in finding his own way around these challenges. Maybe that's one of the jobs of an older therapist, besides anything else that clients ask for during sessions—to show them what it's like to be a well-adjusted and highly functioning elder. It is the kind of thing that people remember for the rest of their lives.

Bring to mind someone you remember from your past who you much admired although they struck you as really, really old. They had an air of equanimity and dignity about them. They seemed remarkably robust and spirited even if they moved a bit slowly. They also provided us templates of what might be possible. In some other cases, we might remember other elderly figures who haunt us to this day and remind us of exactly what we *don't* wish to become. They were object lessons of the dangers we might face someday—to become ornery, rigid, or crippled emotionally.

WHEN IT'S TIME TO QUIT

It seems there was some denial on the part of some of therapists, although we mentioned earlier they said they were more scrupulously honest and self-aware about their aging limitations. Half the sample of therapists we interviewed, most older than 70 years of age, claimed they hadn't notice any differences in their retention of information or ability to remember client material. We suspect an alternative hypothesis would be that some of their memories are so bad they can't recall what they forgot! Anyone older than 60 who has not noticed how much more challenging it is to remember names and little details is living in a bubble of self-deception.

A practicing therapist in his 80s addressed the ethical questions related to his diminished abilities, distinguishing between inner versus outer limitations, those that are actually experienced and should be overlooked versus those imposed by society. He makes a point to check this out with clients during sessions, asking them about how they feel about his advanced age. He reports that most of them are delighted to work with someone with so much experience, but of course this could be part of his own denial.

During the first systematic survey of how older therapists deal with changes associated with aging and impending retirement, Guy, Stark, Poelstra, and Souder (1987) were interested in discovering some of the challenges faced during this stage of career and life. Half of those surveyed planned on retiring by the age of 70—and this questionnaire was distributed 30 years ago. Speaking for the older generation of therapists, Carl Rogers (1980a, 1980b) found that advanced age produced an increase in patience, caring, and acceptance. But, how does one know when you've hung on too long—to the point where some degree of impairment is evident? You forget the names of your clients and family members. You can't recall the details of their history or case. You repeat the same stories over and over again. You become tired or bored much more easily. Maybe you can't even hear what your clients are saying some of the time. Clearly, this interferes with professional effectiveness. And yet we rely on the individual to decide when enough is enough and it's time to quit.

Depression was also mentioned as a frequent issue, less a "mournful refrain" than a reality-based assessment of personal limitations and diminished time. One 60-year-old therapist mentioned the discouraging idea that you realize that the most thrilling experiences of your life are already over, leaving you resigned to whatever is left. Yikes, that *does* sound depressing! And we don't necessarily disagree with that take on things even if one can't help but feel depressed at times with the prospect of infirmity and death becoming a closer reality. Yet there are many of us who don't hit their stride, or enjoy their best adventures, until after 60 and beyond. The new experiences of grandparenting, of being a mentor and sage for younger professionals, are all fulfilling in ways that are unmatched. And with the possibility of more discretionary time, there are new opportunities for adventures that had not been possible previously. This can include travel, but also fulfilling lifelong dreams to write a book, follow an interest, or learn a new skill.

All in all, the vast majority of older therapists in Tallmer's study felt that one of their most important roles was to become a model of successful aging. They felt that growing older has been a positive experience, one that has taught them how to limit their personal ambition in favor of deeper immersion in present moments. They were able to see things in a broader perspective, not take things so seriously and personally, and lessen their competitive drive, which made work and life far more enjoyable.

As a general rule, therapists tend to work longer than most other professionals because of the relatively low demand on physical ability. Fieldsteel (2011) surveyed elderly colleagues, most of them in their 70s and 80s, and none of them had immediate plans to hang up their shingle and retire. One respondent, when queried, replied, "You must be very depressed to even think of such a question. Perhaps you should go back into therapy." Another older gentleman in his 80s said quite seriously, "Ours is a wonderful profession; we can go on forever" (p. 12).

It would be interesting to interview their clients and officemates as well to determine whether they assess the same judgment that their effectiveness still operates at high levels. It begs the question: At what point is it time to accept that aging significantly compromises one's ability to function competently? We are not suggesting a mandatory retirement age, but rather agreeing with Fieldsteel that we have ethical obligations to our clients and the profession to assess our capabilities honestly—and if we can't do so ourselves, then to listen to the feedback from others.

With that said, clients may struggle to talk about some issues with an older therapist, particularly sex; at the very least, erotic transferences are far less likely. Whether it is easier or more embarrassing to talk about such feelings to an older therapist, we have to acknowledge that age differences would certainly have some effect. Freud once complained to a resistant patient who was not getting on board with the expected transference, "You do not think it is worth your

JON: IS IT TIME TO QUIT?

I wish people would quit asking me when I'm going to quit practicing and enjoy retirement. I'm 70 years old and have already been written off as a dead man several times. Between surgeries, chemotherapy, stem cell transplants, blood infusions, antibiotics, it is a wonder of modern science that I am still breathing. I suppose that's why people keep asking me why I'm still working. I almost have to apologize for still wanting to help people, still serving others.

I was forcibly retired from my university position but it feels I have so much left to do, so much to say. I accepted another job so I can start over again because I feel like I'm finally just hitting my stride.

while to love an old man." This feeling was echoed by Chessick (2013, p. 77), who had a similar experience when one of his patients admitted to him, "How can anyone be excited about an old-man analyst?"

Now that's gotta hurt.

In talking further about other things he noticed are different now that he is older, Chessick was sometimes accused by clients of being senile every time he forgot some detail that was considered important. Granted this was likely more about the client's narcissism, but it still represents an age-appropriate hypothesis of slippage—and it also stings.

Accepting reality, and teaching the importance of doing so, is part of our job description. Our clients are often in denial, if not delusional, about their weaknesses and dysfunctional behavior. They consistently misjudge their capabilities, both their strengths as well as weaknesses. They don't often have the most accurate picture of how they are perceived by others, nor are they clear-headed about their impact. If one of our tasks is to help them to collect more accurate data, as well as to provide our own honest feedback, then we would be more than a little hypocritical to avoid doing so for ourselves. Unless we are scrupulously frank with ourselves about what we can't do any longer, we are doomed to repeat the same lapses of judgment.

As her body ages and has become less resilient, Sands (2009) has worked hard to make sure she does what is needed to remain in the best condition: "I must continually learn anew how to self-regulate according to my particular (and changing) needs. All this has helped me become more adept at helping my patients respect and manage their unique bodily and emotional requirements" (p. 166). This is a particularly good example of how successful adjustment to our own aging process helps us to become better at teaching these attitudes and skills to our clients.

WISDOM ACCUMULATED FROM WORK WITH CLIENTS

A therapist in his 70s looks back on his life and career, reflecting on what he's learned from his clients (Geller, 2014). Ever since he completed graduate school so many years ago, he has judged the quality of his relationships with friends and family members based on the same standards and ideals he has set for the intimate connections with his clients. Although he was not able to live up to the impossible goal, he feels appreciative of that ambitious journey. "As my loving wife, Ruth, recently put it," he relates, 'There are times that I wished I was one of your patients so that I could reap the benefits of your patience, kindness, and empathy.' " So true.

Of course we have learned from doing therapeutic work that we can set high expectations for ourselves, try to live up to our ideal standards, and still feel grateful for the continued growth and learning that occurs as long as we keep listening and learning from our clients. Master therapists have, after all, not only attained a lifetime of expertise and wisdom, but they also have learned to be forgiving of our lapses and failures This is a subject that has long fascinated us because of the gifts we have both received as a result of doing this work for a long, long time.

CHAPTER 4
Aging Losses—and Gains

You can live to be a hundred if you give up all the things that make you want to live to be a hundred.

Woody Allen, Comedian and Filmmaker

"Delta 1087, radar contact 18 miles southwest of the Manteca VOR. Maintain 13,000. Turn left heading 2-5-0. Descend and maintain flight level 1-0,000. Cactus 559."

Derek's eyes are glued to the screen while he chomps three sticks of gum that substitute for the chewing tobacco he's trying to quit. If you looked over his shoulder it would appear as if he's playing a video game, but at his ripe age of 53 you would have to reconsider. In fact, he is an air traffic controller and he is concentrating with such intensity that it seems like he's in another world. He is doing his best to keep the little dots spaced at appropriate distances, each one representing a landing aircraft that must be kept miles apart on its approach. Derek spends two consecutive hours staring at the screen, grabbing coffee and something from the snack machine during a 15-minute break, before jumping inside the screen once again.

One would expect that air traffic controllers would have significant trouble as they age, given the critical importance of memory, visual and spatial acuity, cognitive processing, and attention span. Indeed, they *do* lose a certain amount of proficiency in these areas, as would be expected for someone 50 years old. Yet, it turns out they are able to compensate for these losses by learning to adapt other cognitive abilities that are strengthened through experience. They still manage to juggle thousands of pieces of data every minute, navigating and managing dozens of aircraft simultaneously, and making sure there are no collisions (Fields, 2012).

YOU WIN A FEW—AND YOU LOSE A FEW

In this chapter we have a chance to look at just how aging impacts therapists and clients, for better or worse. With aging there are many losses, often irreversible, but also some significant benefits that provide a number of advantages.

In her 80s, Scott-Maxwell (1968) reflected on the meaning of her advanced age, lamenting that she may appear as "wreckage" on the outside but that did not diminish "the flame with a wild life" that was burning brightly on the inside. Yet it feels sad for her to lose so much. "It has taken me all the time I've had to become myself, yet now that I am old, there are times when I feel I am barely here, no room for me at all" (p. 76). She feels invisible, which is so often the case when people feel like they have lost so much of themselves.

Yet, as we well know, losses and gains are often intimately connected, and not necessarily desirable or unwelcome. Loss can lead to freedom and liberation whereas gains by bring additional burdens and responsibility. When we let go of something—a position, commitment, or role—we make room for something else, perhaps a new adventure.

Tom talked about how he was forced to retire as a pilot for one of the major airlines because of his age, but he didn't seem that disappointed. He had already traveled the world and now was looking forward to spending more time at home. He had been in constant motion most of his life, so he was looking forward to remaining still—literally grounded. During the 10 years since retirement, he has not set foot on a plane nor traveled outside a three-county area. He has taken up woodworking and spends most of his time fashioning pens, bowls, and whatever else he can sell in local art and trinket stores. His life has taken a 180-degree turn; he has created new and very different kinds of life adventures. Although many people cannot wait until they retire to be able to travel, Tom could not wait to remain at home.

We don't wish to overromanticize the gains associated with aging because there's little doubt that physiological changes can present a depressing picture indeed. People lose one-third of their teeth by age 60, and half of those older than 85 don't have any teeth left whatsoever. Bones soften as arteries harden. Muscle mass begins to decline every year after age 30. Hair pigment cells become depleted, as does skin elasticity.

Although some gradual vision degeneration is a normal and expected part of aging, more than two million elderly Americans lose much of their eyesight suddenly to macular degeneration (Neighmond, 2014). This produces a cascade of other catastrophic losses in that the afflicted can no longer read, watch television, drive, or cook. They become fearful and isolated, unable to read nonverbal behavior in others. Understandably, they often become seriously depressed.

We mention this as one example of loss because the therapeutic intervention is often more practical and problem solving than the ways we usually think about our jobs. The preferred strategy often involves addressing specific limitations with alternative solutions. Someone who loves to cook might have recipes transposed to exaggerated large print, with one ingredient on each page. Someone who has become reclusive, fearful, and isolated, would be helped to schedule specific "play dates" at accessible locations and conveniently arranged times. It's all about planning and circumventing the limitations.

A TIME OF LOSSES AND TOO MANY CHANGES

There are so many changes associated with aging, many of which are visible every time you glance in the mirror or observe the ways your eating and sleeping patterns are no longer what they once were. There is decreased stamina and energy, just as there are more noticeable aches and pains. Social networks shrink, as does the size of your bladder and physical height. Sensory acuity is compromised in all kinds of little ways that affect sight, touch, hearing, taste, and smell. The immune system, body composition, appearance, and every other organ system are affected in some way, leading to chronic health conditions such as arthritis, hypertension, diabetes, and osteoporosis (Masoro & Austad, 2010). Cognitive processing is slowed along with working short-term, working, and episodic memory. Although dementia is relatively rare (less than 5% before age 80) information processing, multitasking, and executive functions are less efficient (Brickman & Stern, 2009; Glisky, 2007). This explains, in part, why older people are less likely to take risks and avoid novelty in favor of what is familiar and habituated. Beliefs have become entrenched and there is less likelihood of altering these attitudes in the face of new evidence.

Old age is a time of losses, not only of physical capabilities, but also the absence of loved ones, friends, colleagues, and family who have relocated or died. It can mean a loss of some degree of independence and financial resources, along with power and authority. It certainly means a progressive decline in cellular functioning from long-term wear and tear (Carstensen, 2011) (Box 4-1).

The realities of many aspects of aging are inevitable and, in most cases, irreversible. The capacity for maximum oxygen uptake is reduced by 10% every decade after your mid 20s; lung capacity declines by a whopping 40% by the age of 70. Muscle mass similarly shrivels by 25% by that age, and bone mass is reduced faster that it can be replaced (Hill, 2005). The degradation trajectory actually steepens further at this point.

It is certainly discouraging, at least at first glance, to consider that your word fluency and mathematical skills peak by age 50 and then begin to decline, and that verbal fluency, inductive reasoning, and spatial orientation can begin this process even earlier. Yet we also know that general knowledge, semantic memory, and executive functions remain relatively intact throughout one's life span. In fact, it is precisely this matured brain, with organized cognitive templates and established patterns, that leads to more effective problem solving and what we

BOX 4-1 LOSSES OF OLD AGE

Physical abilities	Vitality and energy
Sensory acuity	Memory
Mobility	Autonomy and independence
Family members	Lifelong friends
Social status	Financial resources
Verbal fluency	Social networks
Social networks	Connection to contemporary culture
Self-worth	Feelings of productivity
Professional identity	Sense of self
Emotional attachments	Illusions of immortality

usually think of as wisdom. This can present some challenges for younger therapists working with older clients because their respective brains operate so differently in the ways they approach problems and attempt to resolve them (Agronin, 2010).

Of course, lifestyle choices have a significant impact on the rate of decline, especially related to exercise, smoking, diet, drug and alcohol consumption, and various behavioral habits. Socioeconomic status matters as well, because those with greater resources have access to better healthcare, living situations, and options.

Many of the changes associated with aging are framed as losses—loss of memory, loss of muscle mass, loss of status, and so on. One therapist, reported in a study by Atkins and Lowenthal (2004), works with elderly clients and noted that the accumulative losses of advanced age are magnified by their sheer number: "Loss of a sense of purpose and loss of role from retirement, loss of the identity they got from their jobs and certainly loss of the active person they used to be, so loss of health, loss of mobility, loss of contact with other people and loss of partners, loss of friends, of people dying around them" (p. 52).

Berthelsdorf (1992) remarked that one of the most distressing aspects of growing old is the loss of one's friends: "In that gathering of memory no one is left to mourn one's own passing" (p. 67). Who remains as a "significant other?" Caregivers? Children and grandchildren and great grandchildren? There is nobody left who really understands what it's like to be of an age.

Growing old may be a gradual, imperceptible process that is barely noticed by our clients because they are aging at the same time, but this is not the case with the consequences of being elderly. Hurwitz (1992) describes what happened when he had a heart attack and then, later, other illnesses. His clients became angry at him for not being as available and responsive as they had come to expect. He, in turn, felt furious at their self-centeredness. Here he was fighting for his health, if not his life, and all the clients seemed to think about was their own narcissistic needs. Later he considered that it is also likely they were upset by his vulnerability and fragility, that he wasn't the infallible, all-knowing, all-powerful, indestructible authority figure who was impervious to the risks of mortal beings.

As his memory began to betray him later in life, Hurwitz (1992) described the ways he would deliberately slow down the pace of his work and his daily life. He had to learn to be patient and accepting of his limitations. He had to develop ways to adjust and compensate for his lapses. In preparing bills he would frequently misspell words or names, enter wrong dates, or make simple arithmetic errors that only seemed to broadcast to clients his problems. So he learned to double-check his work more often, something he'd never had to do before. He became quick to acknowledge mistakes, apologize for them, and move on. He learned to become more forgiving of himself, which, as it turns out, is excellent modeling for clients who come to us as such harsh self-critics.

RULES AND EXCEPTIONS

As we've mentioned, not all memory processes become compromised and degenerate with age. Although it is true that it becomes harder to remember names or to access certain words or numbers, to manage multiple tasks at the same time, other systems such as pattern recognition not only remain intact but also operate at peak levels. "The young man knows the rules," Oliver Wendell Holmes observed, "but the old man knows the exceptions." It is that awareness of exceptions to the rules that helps compensate for the very real losses.

As memory begins to slip, older therapists often learn to accept these changes as part of the process. One older therapist with memory challenges calmly announced to his students in the classroom or clients in the consulting room that he had so much to remember that his retrieval system couldn't be expected to keep up with the vast amount of knowledge at this disposal. He didn't panic or worry, but vowed to share whatever was misplaced in a few minutes or later. And if the data or story still remained elusive, he told clients or students that he would just e-mail it later. The important thing is that he didn't overreact, or even become unduly self-critical; he just accepted his new reality and adapted accordingly. Of course, it helps that he is constantly reassured by others that, even being forgetful, he still knows more than almost anyone else. He knows the rules, but also so many more exceptions to those standard expectations.

From age 20 onward, there are definite changes that take place in the reduction of brain volume. By 40, the cortex shrinks noticeably. The hippocampus is reduced in size. The frontal lobes operate less efficiently, leading to increased distractibility and habitual rather than measured reactions to situations (cognitive inflexibility). Neuronal connections become less reliable as dendrites shorten and neurotransmitters such as dopamine and serotonin become depleted. The hormones and proteins largely responsible for repairing brain cells or growing new ones are also less available. Blood flow to the brain diminishes. Sensory systems become less sensitive and responsive. Reaction times slow down. Mental processes lose some steam as well.

And yet these alterations in brain structure and chemistry do not necessarily lead to decline. It may take longer for older people to remember certain words, but that's, in part, because they know more of them than those who are younger. This may explain why, for example, that crossword puzzle experts continue to improve their skills well into old age (Salthouse, 2012).

Significant losses are consistently reported in people older than 50 related to episodic memory (Where did I park my car?), source memory (Where did I read that?), and flashbulb memory (Where was I when I got the news about the job?). Yet there is relatively little loss experienced in verbal (vocabulary and semantics) or procedural (driving a car, operating a device) memory. Among the everyday memory tasks about which older people often complain, there are a few areas that are most affected with aging—most of them already familiar to anyone older than 50. These include forgetting where things are placed, retrieving the right word in a sentence, and remembering names and faces. A fourth example that used to be reported frequently but is now no longer relevant involves remembering phone numbers; but, of course, nowadays *nobody* remembers phone numbers because mobile devices do that for us.

Goldberg (2005), a neuropsychologist who studies the cognitive changes that take place during aging, reflected on what he noticed about his own capabilities when he turned 60, concluding that his mind was neither stronger nor weaker than it had been throughout his life. He noticed that he was no longer a whiz at solving new problems any longer as much as he could recognize familiar patterns he'd encountered previously; his brain seemed to come to solutions automatically and intuitively without conscious thought. "I am not nearly as good at laborious, grinding, focused mental computations; but then again I do not experience the need to resort to them nearly as often" (p. 8–9). And that is Goldberg's main thesis related to how the aging brain adapts to its changes—by relying on quite different mental functions that become strengthened with age and experience.

THE BENEFITS AND GAINS ASSOCIATED WITH GROWING OLDER

There is one thing we know about the aging experience: loss is a certainty. If one lives long enough, there will be loss of friends, opportunities, optimal functioning, memory, energy, choices, and eventually life itself. And unless there is a simultaneous plane or car crash, there is likelihood that one partner will die before the other. Such losses, with their accompanying bereavement and necessary adjustments, become fertile areas to explore in therapy. Yet the vast majority of surviving spouses eventually recover quite well on their own, even with the devastating loss of their life partner (Bonnano, Wortman, & Neese, 2004).

Characteristic of the "resilient responders" was their ability to engage in active coping strategies for their grief, specifically focusing on their most positive memories. Second, they facilitated their own recovery and adjustment by reaching beyond previous lifestyle patterns, experimenting with new options and developing new interests.

Kitra was extremely close to her husband for more than 40 years, after which he slowly died of cancer during the course of a year. This transition gave her time to consider what her life would be like when she was alone. Previously in their relationship, she had been content to go along with her husband's preferences. They lived a rather austere life, primarily saving money to distribute to their children. But, when Kitra realized that, for the first time in her life, she would have to make her own choices for the future, she decided to pursue interests that had long fascinated her: traveling the world, moving to a different part of town. She negotiated very different relationships with her children than they had been used to previously, and she began to structure a very independent lifestyle although she was in her mid 80s.

Kitra's situation, however, was possible because of several factors that are not always present. First, she had the financial means to live a comfortable life and make choices that are not possible for those who are struggling. Second, she enjoyed a very close relationship with her husband; it would appear that those who have problematic marriages are more likely to fall into the category of "chronic grievers" because of issues that were never resolved while their partner was alive. It is for this reason that the preexisting condition of a marriage and a client's functioning have a lot to do with how successfully he or she copes with losses.

From an aging therapist's perspective, Martha Kirkpatrick (1992) reflected on the wisdom she has gained spending a lifetime in her profession. She modestly admitted that she may have only been an adequate practitioner—better than some, worse than others—but she also found her unique voice. She found that it was one of the gifts of age that she was no longer intimidated by anyone, nor was she filled with envy toward those who were younger.

As satisfied as she might have felt by this sense of grounding, Kirkpatrick is also mourning the loss of one of her most prized possessions: her near photographic memory. Now she forgets some of the details of her sessions, even the names of her clients and their family members, the names of almost anything—words, places, books, movies.

Yet, what is she to do? She's too old to change professions and she still feels too young to quit. Ultimately, she accepts that her role in life is to assemble and integrate the disparate pieces of herself. She is teaching herself to let go of ambition and drive, her attachment to remaining so productive, and instead focuses on speaking her voice more clearly.

There are indeed some distinct benefits of reaching a certain position in the profession as a result of experience and seniority. Jerry Corey, who we mentioned in the previous chapter, really enjoys the attention and respect he receives whenever he attends a conference. "I must admit that it feels affirming to be recognized and appreciated by so many professionals, many of whom I have not met before. Many of these individuals go out of their way to talk with me, or to ask to take a picture with me, and tell me how they have been influenced by my work."

Corey is reluctant to say that this attention is a function of his age, but rather the result from all his hard work throughout the years. Indeed, people are surprised at his self-discipline related to writing—how he can produce so many books. But in some ways, he is just as proud of the commitment involved in taking care of himself so he remains so engaged and energetic.

"People are always surprised when I tell them that I exercise for several hours every day, rain or shine, no matter where I am. This includes walking, hiking, biking, but I also do Pilates and stretching." He is also rather strict about when and how he eats and sleeps, feeling a sense of control over his remarkably good health.

When asked about the greatest gifts and advantages of being an elder in the field, he points to differences in opportunities and responsibilities than when he was younger. "In earlier years, when I was in my 30s and 40s, I was so busy with my teaching, writing, counseling, traveling, plus taking care of my family. It didn't feel like I had many choices." He's not saying that he didn't *have* choices, just that it didn't feel like it.

Corey is still engaged in all these activities, but now at a much more moderate and selective pace. It feels like now he can choose what he wants to do in ways that these options didn't seem as possible earlier in life. This allows him more time to reflect on what he's doing, what he's been doing his whole life, and try to put it in some meaningful perspective. Being existentially inclined helps with this task, and reminds us once again of the privileges we enjoy being a part of the therapist guild. We have spent our whole lives helping others to look deeply at life's most important questions, and we prepared ourselves to do the same in our own lives.

Talking about some of these issues stirred things up for Corey. Soon after the thoughts expressed earlier, he had a vivid dream: "I am at a conference and I walk into a room and someone is presenting something in an experiential way. I recall being a bit critical of what he was doing. Then I walk into a large room with elevated chairs [theater style] and someone asks me to present something since the audience is sitting there and the speaker didn't show up. I am talking to them about group therapy and then, while I'm in mid-sentence, a whole bunch of people get up together and leave. I am standing there thinking that maybe they needed to go to another event. There are just three people still in the audience and they tell me how rude it is that so many people got up and left!"

After mentioning the dream to his wife, Marianne, she suggested that the three people left in the audience might have included her and their two daughters. So that gets him wondering: "Maybe I'm anxious, after all, that people don't care what I have to say anymore. That is definitely one of my fears as an elder."

JEFFREY: WHO ARE WE KIDDING?

I was just reading a passage in one of the hundreds of books we've consulted on "positive" or "successful" or "optimal" aging. The author was talking about how invigorating and rewarding being older is, how wise and experienced we've become, how fortunate older people are to have attained such a position in life.

No matter how we romanticize aging, it sometimes sucks. There are aches and pains that crop up out of nowhere. I can measure my deterioration every year by the times I run in 10-kilometer races: I lose about 15 seconds or more each year.

I know. I know. Just because I'm moving slower doesn't mean I'm enjoying the experience any less (if it could be said that running a race is enjoyable). But I find the overidealizing of aging to be disingenuous. Who wouldn't, if given the opportunity, take an elixir that promises eternal youth? Who would ever wish on themselves the slow, progressive losses of functioning? Who would want to see their age-mates fall into disability or death? Who would want to look in a mirror and see someone they barely recognize any longer?

I'm just trying to be really honest here. Obviously, we have little choice in the matter of when we age, but of course we do choose *how* we age, and how we feel about the situation.

ADAPTING TO CHANGES

Bermann (2009) had been dyeing her hair and disguising her advancing age for some time, although she was quite aware that some of these choices were both unhealthy and incongruent with her values of authenticity. She realized that being an elder provided her with a degree of experience, confidence, security, and wisdom that she had not known previously. She was now in a better position to challenge some of her choices and delve deeply into areas where others fear to tread. She had been rejecting and denying her age, as well as avoiding the vulnerabilities with youth left behind. "I've been avoiding my own reactions to my aging each day as I look in the mirror, and also avoiding the negative judgments of aging women in our culture as I navigate the world" (Bermann, 2009, p. 271).

When she embraced the gifts of her experience, Bermann found that she was able to sit with her clients with much greater stillness and serenity than ever before. She noticed that she had become quieter and less controlling as she matured as a therapist.

As we've mentioned, there are a number of things that don't change with age—notably, one's level of self-esteem and life satisfaction that, in most cases, actually improves (Carstensen & Hartel, 2006). This may be related in part to more modest expectations, but they still signal some of the benefits enjoyed by older people. Because they often expect less from therapy, or anything else, it is far easier to deliver a satisfying outcome. With more realistic views of what is possible, this is one reason why older adults are less prone to depression and anxiety than their younger counterparts, and they are much more emotionally stable (Charles & Cartensen, 2010; Gum, King-Kallimanis, & Kohn, 2009).

There are all kinds of evidence that older people are actually far better at managing and stabilizing emotions, staying on an even keel, and demonstrating better self-control. They are less likely to experience or express anger or act impulsively (Fields, 2012). Obviously, this is a tremendous advantage when doing psychotherapy.

In surveys of people older than the age of 75, they consistently say they don't much feel old at all; they say they feel at least 10 to 20 years younger than their actual age. The majority of them also look back on their lives and feel quite satisfied with the way things have turned out. Among those who have survived past 85, only 1 in 100 say their life turned out worse than they expected. Even with inevitable financial problems, illnesses, and sensory and memory losses, the vast majority also report they are quite happy, as much so as any other stage in life. In addition, what makes them happy are essentially the same factors valued at any other time—a few good friends, reasonably good health, and a degree of financial security (Taylor, 2009). There were also a few surprises in this study by the Pew Research Center—notably, being married or not didn't seem to predict happiness in old age, which is good thing considering the number of them who are widowed. Second, an increasing number of them who may say they are "retired" are still working at least part-time in some employment or volunteer position. It is clear that the meaning of being old has changed significantly in recent years, requiring new, adjusted perceptions of this life stage.

HELPING OTHERS (AND OURSELVES) DEAL WITH LOSSES

Therapists are certainly well aware that attitudes and beliefs play a critical role in how people deal with their experiences, especially with regard to losses, disappointments, and even traumatic events. And so it is the case that how older clients deal with the predictable and inevitable changes associated with aging depends very much on their subjective interpretations, and varies tremendously from individual to individual.

"I used to be so frustrated that I couldn't hear as well as I used to," one man in his 60s mentioned to his therapist. "It must have been all those rock concerts I attended in college, or maybe I've had the volume turned up too loud listening to my favorite songs." He shrugged, but then thoughtfully added the way he has adjusted his thinking.

"Sure, it is sometimes annoying that I become impatient with my wife because it seems like she talks so softly, but then I realized that there have been some advantages as well." He is referring to how *all* sounds have become muted to his ears; it used to drive him crazy to hear dogs barking in the neighborhood or people talking in movie theaters. He was easily distracted by intrusive sounds and noises, claiming that his brain could focus only on one thing at a time, but now he found the volume of the world "blissfully" turned down and he can concentrate better when reading or working on a project.

It is such adaptation and attitudinal adjustments that Vaillant (2007) found so critical in his long-term study of successful aging. He discovered that those most satisfied during later life weren't just interested in coping with losses and dealing with struggles, but rather that they retained a capacity for "sustained joy." He studied more than 800 individuals during the course of their lifetimes, especially with regard to how they handled age-related changes, and found that those who were happiest and most satisfied had managed to develop flexible and optimistic outlooks in dealing with their challenges. They focused on their current relationships as much as possible instead of dwelling on those from the past. They practiced forgiveness and gratitude rather than holding on to resentments and disappointments. They maintained a sense of humor that helped them to moderate the pain of losses. And most critically, Vaillant identified that subjective assessment of health trumped their actual objective physical condition. Despite any disabilities or physical disintegration, they found a measure of peace and acceptance with things outside of their control.

In addition to any usual and customary assessment questions that might be included, we must create a more expansive view of client functioning in terms of essential goals and significant priorities. We have thus restructured our intake profile to include asking questions that emphasize strengths and resources as much as losses and problems:

- What do you consider to be the most important things in your life right now?
- List the five best things about you and your life right now.

- What have you noticed are the most significant changes that you've experienced in recent years, for better or worse?
- What are some things going on in your life that sap your energy or make things difficult for you that you would like to eliminate?
- What could we do together that would help you to become more optimistic and hopeful about the future?

In a study of how older people adapt and accommodate to the losses they experience, Dockendorff (2014) acknowledges that, although they frequently make reference to diminished capacity, increased fatigue, deteriorating health, and aches and pains, successful coping seemed to be related to several strategies—most notably, acceptance of what can no longer be. Rather than whining and complaining about how things are different, high-functioning individuals are able to deal with the realities of their situation, especially related to aspects that were no longer within their power. One 68-year-old woman who struggles with fatigue and chronic stiffness said, "I have tried to maintain an attitude of not fighting Parkinson's, but instead, of learning from the disease" (p. 368). Second, they develop increased self-reliance. With reduced social support, adaptation often took the form of increased personal resolve, as described by an 83-year-old woman who has lost many of her friends and family members: "I don't think they know the pain that I've felt because I've never said anything; quietly, I just keep going" (p. 369). The central theme of Dockendorff's study is that successful adaptors to loss were realistic with themselves about what they could do and couldn't do, and they made the best of their situation instead of dwelling on the way things used to be.

Successful adaptation to any loss, whether of a loved one, bodily function, or youth, is obviously characterized by adjusting goals and being far more selective. With aging, it is critical that choices be prioritized because there is less time, and fewer resources and energy. Older people must be helped to figure out what is truly most important to them, and to focus efforts on those tasks and activities, and invest in particular relationships, rather than trying to cover too much territory. This is framed by therapists, not as a form of "sacrifice," but rather as "optimization." Finally, clients must be helped to compensate for their changes and losses by finding other means by which to satisfy the same or similar needs. One example of how an older person might combine these strategies is mentioned by Baltes, Lindenberger, and Staudinger (1998) in the case of concert pianist Arthur Rubinstein. By the time the great musician had reached the age of 80, he was still playing on stage and still bringing audiences to their feet with his virtuoso performances. When asked how it was possible that he could still maintain such a high level of excellence in his music, Rubenstein mentioned several strategies that were consistent with the points just raised. First, he concentrated on mastering a smaller repertoire of pieces that allowed him to focus on a more manageable task. Second, he learned to adapt his practice schedule so that he worked on the pieces more often to compensate for memory losses. Third, he developed new techniques to cover for the slower speed of his hands by deliberately slowing down some of the more *allegro* segments to make the parts that came afterward appear to be so much faster.

The same adjustments must be made when older therapists learn to compensate for their reduced speed of mental processing, or flagging stamina, by evolving other ways to remain alert and focused. Likewise, therapists must also learn to adjust expectations and actions to match the capabilities of their older clients. Mary Pipher (1999), now an elderly therapist herself, remembers the adaptations she would make when visiting older clients, and doing so with patience and equanimity: "I learned to let the phone ring fifteen times. I learned to wait at doors five minutes after I rang the bell. I had to slow down with the old. Their conversation was less linear, and there are pauses and repetitions. Points are made via stories; memories lead to more memories" (Pipher, 1999, p. 27).

AGING OPTIMALLY

It is time for us to take the lead to reframe what it means to be old, following what Hill (2005) has called "positive" or "optimal aging," even if only 10% of us ever attain that ideal. This is not a state of being that is based on physical age (whether 60 or 90), or even physical condition (whether healthy, disabled, or in chronic pain), but rather a state of mind and chosen attitude. Adapting the work of Seligman and Csikszentmihalyi (2000), Hill describes that state of exceptional well-being among the elderly as characterized by the following attributes:

- Hope and optimism for the future
- Accommodative coping with physical changes
- Continued growth, learning, and personal development
- Acceptance of losses without isolation
- Active social engagement and intimate relationships
- Maintenance and improvement of health and physical functioning
- Appropriate adjustment of goals and priorities
- Forgiveness of past slights, injustices, and wounds
- Setting of limits that are age appropriate

Most of these factors can be reduced to one essential and critical strategy, and that involves developing maximum flexibility in a variety of ways. First of all, one must be honest with oneself about what can and can't be done within realistic parameters. This means adjusting goals and priorities, staying within limits to avoid injury and avoiding frustration, and yet still striving for new learning and growth to keep oneself active and engaged.

Therapists are ideally positioned to help older people to assess realistically what is within their capacity, to work through unresolved issues, and find greater meaning in what is within one's grasp. This often does not take place without some kind of professional intervention to confront distortions and denial. Learning to accept what we can't change, and to change what we can, has been a part of all of the other life stages; this one is no different.

Fred has been living with cancer for many years. He is in his mid 70s and has spent several years with pain, confusion, and fear as the cancer metastasized to his bladder and spine. Fred shares, "It's difficult for us to see that life is truly wonderful and full of change and challenges, and to remember that learning to see and share that beauty with others is rewarding. It's important to understand that we need to work at being an adult or senior and that learning doesn't stop. That we can contribute in our community in many ways to keep it beautiful, clean, and healthy. When we do participate, it contributes to our own health and well-being."

Taking Fred's advice, we move on to the ways that a lifetime of experience can provide a number of shortcuts and expedient modes of operating that capitalize on the gifts that aging offers.

CHAPTER 5

Tricks of the Trade

What Experience Teaches Us

Looking back it seems to me that I was clueless until I was about 50 years old.
Nora Ephron, Author

"I've been teaching, supervising, and doing therapy for longer than I can remember," a therapist in his mid 60s noted, "and remembering is actually the biggest problem. I could instantly remember names of students. I could recall every detail of a session, hardly needing to write anything down."

This therapist was initially so frustrated because he considered memory to be his greatest asset. Memory is what allows us to make connections between seemingly unrelated pieces of a client's life. Memory is what helps us to build intimacy in relationships because of the ways we can demonstrate how closely and carefully we listen.

"I actually thought about just packing it in, deciding I just couldn't do this work anymore," the therapist added. "But then I figured that young people today can't remember much of anything because they are so dependent on technology. They can't remember phone numbers because they never actually call them. They don't need to hardly memorize anything because they can just instantly look it up online. That kind of reminded me that I could compensate as well if I just made some adjustments in the way I do things and stop whining about how things used to be different when I was younger."

At first this therapist was self-conscious about the changes he introduced into his work. He took photos of his students and made flash cards with their names, flipping through them before each class. He started taking notes during sessions so he could hold on to details that would otherwise slip through his attention. He started spacing out sessions during the day to give him more time to recover. He even reduced the time of sessions from 50 minutes to 45 minutes so he had breaks to use the bathroom frequently. All in all, it wasn't so much that that the quality of his work suffered as it just changed in significant ways—or rather he made necessary adjustments that helped him to function optimally.

LESSONS FROM THE OLDEST OLD

Aging well is, above all else, about adaptation. Whether we are talking about older people in general, or older therapists in particular, life experience provides a number of important lessons that, if honored, lead to greater wisdom and success in almost any enterprise. Loe (2011) was especially interested in what choices and strategies the "oldest old" make—their tricks of the trade so to speak—that were most helpful in later life. She studied the ways that 30 people in their 80s and 90s, living alone and independently, managed to lead extraordinarily satisfying and meaningful lives. This wasn't a truly representative sample, considering that almost all the participants in the study were white and native born, but it nevertheless highlighted some important lessons that were consistent in their stories. These dozen lessons are instructive not only for understanding better what seems to be most helpful in later life, but also they provide us with goals we might wish to incorporate in our own work and lives.

1. They continued doing the things that gave them pleasure and satisfaction throughout their lives. This might have been walking in their neighborhood, following their favorite sports teams, watching game shows, volunteering in a hospital, or remaining active in their congregations.
2. They redesigned their living spaces to make it easier for them to take care of themselves without assistance. That is one crucial reason why they were able to maintain an independent life. They organized their living quarters for easy access to the TV remote, refrigerator, and phone. They improved the lighting. They designed their bathrooms to be handicap accessible. They reduced the amount of daily living space to make things more manageable, which leads to the next lesson.
3. They lived in moderation. They found it far easier to simplify their lives as much as possible. They lived with less, which both reduced their financial burden and workload. They avoided necessary risks such as walking on icy sidewalks or eating things they knew would upset their equilibrium.
4. They learned to enjoy their own company. Although older adults living on their own might appear lonely and isolated we know this is usually not the case. Many older people quite enjoy and prefer their own company, and find their daily routines to be comfortable and grounding. They immerse themselves in books, TV shows, cooking, puzzles and games, gardening, naps, or creative activities.

5. They are not afraid to ask for help when they need it. They are practical and realistic about what they can't handle on their own, respecting their limits. If family members or neighbors are not available as resources, then they make proactive arrangements for deliveries, errands, transportation, and medical consultations.
6. Although they are living alone, they also connect with others on a regular basis and on their own terms. Apart from family gatherings, they also find it important to spend time with peers, playing cards or scrabble, joining a book club, participating in water aerobics, or hanging out at a community center.
7. They've kept a sense of humor. They consider laughter and fun a part of their lives. They describe themselves as "jokesters," "smartasses," "happy-go-lucky." They use humor as a way to deal with hardships.
8. They have a "job." This doesn't mean they go to work (although they might!). They have responsibilities they take seriously, whether checking on a neighbor, taking care of children or pets, committing to a cause, mentoring family members, or providing emotional support to others.
9. They've created their own "family." In addition to any biological relatives, they also form "tribes" for mutual support. They "adopt" people into multigenerational family units, including friends, neighbors, caregivers, pets, and members of their congregation.
10. They feel loved. Affection is important to them, both showing love to others and receiving it. Touch and hugs are valued.
11. They are adaptable and resilient. They recover from disappointments, setbacks, losses, disabilities, and body changes by making necessary adjustments. They persevere despite the obstacles they face. Even with a number of physical limitations, even chronic pain, they still find ways to do what they value most.
12. They accept and prepare for death. They acknowledge they have little time left, so they want to make the most of their opportunities. They reflect on what it means to have a "good death"—one with dignity and a certain feeling of control over some aspects of the experience.

The lifestyle choices mentioned in this study would appear to be useful with regard to any other stage in life, even if they take on greater importance as clients (and therapists) grow older. It is also curious how, regardless of chronological age, some people remain young in spirit whereas others have always seemed to be old way beyond their years.

GENERATIVITY AND A LIFE'S WORK

Perhaps the most significant secret of older people who continue to lead meaningful and productive lives, whether as therapists or members of any other professional group, is they have figured out how to remain engaged and active in their daily life. It's important to remember that the whole concept of "retirement" is a relatively recent phenomenon in human existence. First of all, before the last century or two people worked until they keeled over since community survival depended on *everyone* pitching in to do their share of tasks, even if only to care for others. The idea of a pension wasn't even "invented" until the Industrial Revolution, and Social Security wasn't introduced until 1935. The idea is that people would devote most of their lives to productive work followed by subsidies that would allow them to enjoy their "golden years" playing golf and bridge. That fantasy didn't actually apply to those who couldn't afford to stop working because of financial challenges, and those who actually enjoyed their work and didn't view it as a burden. Nevertheless, changes during the past decade as a result of the Great Recession and adult children moving back home have put an added incentive for older people to continue working way beyond the traditional retirement age of 65. When we consider that many people will live well into their 90s, it begs the question of what sort of meaningful activities they will engage in for two or three decades of active existence.

Moody and Sasser (2015) question whether the whole concept of retirement is even obsolete. They note that more people are choosing—or being required—to remain in the labor force. Older women, in particular, are entering the workforce with increasing frequency, in some cases because of economic necessity but in other instances because they are finally freed from previous obligations to do some things they had always wanted to pursue.

This presents some intriguing new issues to explore in therapy with older clients (and ourselves!): discussing ways they might wish to remain productive during this stage of life, whether through volunteering, paid employment, radical career changes, social commitments, or family responsibilities. On the other hand, there have been some myths circulating about the consequences of retirement—that supposedly it is bad for one's health and leads to an inevitable decline toward inactivity and depression. It turns out there is little, if any, evidence for this belief, and although more and more people are expressing a distinct preference for working longer, others make different choices and do just as well.

There are distinct differences among therapists approaching traditional retirement age. Some choose to work until they drop (or fall asleep in their chair) whereas others look forward to alternative options in their last years of practice. Among those we interviewed for this project, we heard a whole assortment of different responses that ranged from some who never wished to see a client again and wanted to get as far away as possible from the profession to others who felt more engaged than ever in their therapeutic work.

After Michael Hoyt retired from active practice for a large mental health organization, he talked to a number of friends and colleagues about how they had adapted to their new lifestyles. They reported to him about ways that their sense of time had changed. Ordinarily our lives are partitioned into 50-minute segments during sessions and then, all of a sudden, there is a sense of freedom related to the pace of daily life. Of course this can also create a sense of anxiety or boredom with all the unstructured time, as well as feelings of being lost. Hoyt remembers meeting someone at a social function and when the person learned he had recently retired asked him, "Oh! Who did you used to be?"

Such questions have forced Hoyt to consider what's next during this stage of life. "One retires *from* something," he muses, "but one also retires *to* something. So, what's next? How about more travel? Maybe the Peace Corps? Attending more lectures or taking classes? Breaking 80 on the golf course? Hanging out with friends? Spending more time with my wife? Writing another book? Opening a private practice? Supervising interns? Hiking with the dog? Reading books? Volunteering? But to do what?"

What indeed?

We've asked the question previously: what use are older people, given their decreased contributions to the community? Until the 1950s it had long been assumed by scientists that menopause had no evolutionary function whatsoever. It turns out that the end of fertility is *not* the end of reproduction. Older members of the community are still very involved in taking care of children and ensuring their survival. Menopause may have developed as a way to protect the survival of the young when human births became more risky and the infants who were more dependent on care (Williams, 1957). This makes clearer why and how human longevity is necessary for our continued survival, and the significant role that older adults (especially grandmothers) play when their active biological reproduction ceases (Hawkes & Coxworth, 2013).

As one example, taking on responsibilities as a mentor and/or grandparent often has a positive impact on the well-being of older people, especially with the dramatic changes that have taken place to enhance the role (Maijala, Uusiautti, & Maatta, 2013). Never before have grandparents been healthier, more active, and better educated. They have access to transportation and technology that now permit virtual daily contact with family members via mobile video devices, which deepen those relationships in ways that have never been possible before.

"Becoming a grandparent changed *everything* for me," related one man who, until the birth of his granddaughter, was still focused mostly on his work. "After she was born, all I could think about was how much I wanted to be with her as much as possible. It was so different than being a parent. I was so much younger and clueless then. I was so concerned with making a living and supporting my family, working long hours. I missed so much of my children growing up. But it feels like I have a second chance to do things right this time. I am so much more patient than I had been in my youth. Sure, I have trouble keeping up with the little tyke swirling around like a typhoon, but it feels like I have even a greater capacity to love in ways that almost shock me."

It is clear from this and other examples that the "older self" is indeed a different person than the being who existed earlier in life. There are some challenges associated with accepting and adapting to these changes, but also some new opportunities.

NEW WAYS OF BEING ONESELF

There is little doubt that the productivity and creativity of the elderly are usually undervalued. They are most often viewed as receivers rather than givers of care, yet one study investigated the contributions they make to their communities in four domains (Wiles & Jayasinha, 2013).

The first included *volunteering.* Many of the older people felt a strong commitment to social justice issues, following through with work on behalf of significant causes. This included helping refugees in the community, working in preschools, or teaching the English language. One retired therapist we know feels useful walking his neighborhood each morning, picking up trash along the way. He works in partnership with another neighbor to take care of a local land conservancy, trimming the wooded area and keeping it free of debris.

Another contribution was *activism.* This involved participating in political causes, lobbying, and attending public meetings—to mention a few possibilities—or taking a leadership role promoting social causes that improve the quality of life for the community. One man in his 70s, who retired from active practice a few years ago, has never felt busier or more satisfied with his life. He works on local and national political campaigns, and he accepted a volunteer position with the organization that advocates and monitors the state pension fund. He also used his knowledge and skills as a therapist and educator to be appointed to the state board of higher education. All of this is in addition to playing on a senior softball team in whatever spare time he has left.

The third commitment was *nurturing.* Beyond grandparenting roles, many older people remain active by supporting their local community. They often view their primary role as sustaining cherished cultural values. Some visit shut-ins through their local churches. Others serve "meals on wheels." Many still help their children and grandchildren in a variety of ways.

Although this study mentioned was conducted in New Zealand with members of the indigenous Maori people, a culture that demonstrates more than the usual respect for elders, it nevertheless highlights the ways that older people remain active and engaged in their communities, as well as feel like productive and useful citizens. Much of the work of counseling elders involves helping them to find meaningful ways to serve others.

Howard Kirschenbaum, after reaching the age of 70, contemplated the next stage of his life and what he wanted to do with the time that was left. Kirschenbaum had spent his whole career as a scholar, faculty member in counseling, and official biographer of Carl Rogers.

"It seems like I've retired in stages," he said. "I've watched others keep on keeping on, and I've admired those figures like Albert Ellis and William Glasser continuing to remain productive until their 90s, but I no longer have that kind of ambition or motivation."

Kirschenbaum paused for moment, carefully considering how best to express what he had been experiencing. "I'm now retired—not by anyone else's choice or even by my own. There was no letter of resignation this time, no announcement, no farewell parties, not even a list of pros and cons culminating in an active decision to retire. I simply finished up what I was working on professionally and didn't begin anything new. It's not that I've firmly decided not to do anything more; if something intriguing comes along—a particular keynote, an interesting consulting request, something that grabs me for one reason or another—I would consider it. But if it doesn't, that's just fine. For now I *feel* retired."

That said, what Kirschenbaum means is that, although he may have retired as a therapist and educator, he now has a renewed interest and energy to pursue other projects that have long interested him, ones that help him to feel active and engaged.

"I may have eased out of one professional life, but I have ramped up my other vocation as the manager of a historical resort." This means there's been no time for an "identity crisis" because he's so busy with his new work, which has been made considerably easier considering that he has devoted most of his research and practice to launching the values clarification movement. "As hard as I worked to become a 'somebody,' I never took it very seriously in the sense of identifying with my professional identity. I know this is a bit of a paradox, but as proud as I've been of my professional accomplishments, they never went to my head. I think I always knew that, in the large scheme of things, my contributions were relatively modest. And over the years, I came to understand increasingly that the quality of my relationships with others and with myself was more important than professional identity or worldly success."

One other reason that Kirschenbaum's transition to "retirement" has been relatively seamless is that he has planned it for so long and has so much he is looking forward to. "I envision the coming years to be very rich—a continuation of a direction I've been moving in for several years—having fewer major responsibilities for projects and more discretionary time to live as I choose on a day-to-day basis. I intend to still make some contributions to the world around me, but also allow lots of time to indulge my own avocational and recreational inclinations."

As for many older professionals, Kirschenbaum experiences time very differently than when he was younger. "I do have a growing sense of mortality—not a morbid one, but a recognition that I'm getting old. Most of the time I don't *feel* old, but sometimes, more and more, I realize that I'm getting old, especially when

I look in the mirror. Therefore, each year ahead seems very precious, contributing to the feeling, the resolve, that it's time to live as I'd like to live, to try a different way of living than how I've done it for most of my adult life."

As mentioned, one of the main subject's of Kirschenbaum's work was to write several biographies about his mentor, Carl Rogers. After turning 75, Rogers (1980b) wrote an essay looking back on the previous decade of his life during a time when most people had already retired, especially during that era. He admitted some physical changes; he could no longer throw a Frisbee without pain in his shoulder or work in the garden as long as he used to. Yet, he still walked four miles most days, and carried his own luggage during his world travels doing 16-day intensive workshops or negotiating peace treaties between nations at war. His work productivity felt as exciting and innovative as ever, even as he traded clinical practice and academia for his new vision in creating the Center for Studies of the Person—"the zaniest, most improbable, and most influential non-organization imaginable" (p. 6).

This nonorganization paralleled his own new discoveries related to "new ways of being myself" (Rogers, 1980b). He began to experiment with new therapeutic structures, what he called "extremely far-out gambles," leading groups in Brazil with 800 people in a circle (12 deep). After what he described as "initial chaos," people began listening to one another and sharing deep feelings.

During his 70s, Rogers became more of a risk-taker than ever. In part, this was the result of feeling the urgency of limited time, but also it was possible because of the support he felt from his team, which gave him courage. It also helped that this was during the 1960s, when "anything goes," and Rogers felt such an affinity for the youth movement's experimentations and rebelliousness. "I am bored by safety and surety," he admitted. "I become bored with myself" (Rogers, 1980b, p. 9). What was most remarkable was that during a time when older people are supposed to be set in their ways, Rogers continued to remain open to new ideas, especially related to "inner space" and the power of intuition.

It was during these last years of his life that Rogers' research and writing took on a different focus and style. He was interested in expanding his ideas to transform schools and education, to promote personal power and freedom for a wider audience beyond therapy. He identified strongly with Abraham Maslow's thinking about aging related to self-actualization. Just as Maslow kept writing until the very end, Rogers intended to do the same as a way to remain engaged and productive.

On a more personal level, Rogers also experienced a number of changes during the last decade of his life. Self-care became a priority. He began to curtail his drinking, spent more time in solitary retreat, and asked for help more often. Intimacy and sexuality opened up for him in new ways, trying to feed his craving for deep sharing. "I am more ready to touch and be touched physically . . . I am more aware of the sensuous side of my life" (Rogers, 1980b, p. 13). He started hugging people a lot more and initiating more physical contact.

Despite the recognition and validation he was receiving for his life's work, Rogers also experienced his fair share of personal struggles. He was a caretaker for his sick and dying wife, which filled him with despair and helplessness. Although he didn't admit to depression and confusion very often, he nevertheless did have some difficulties that he mostly kept hidden.

Although Kirschenbaum found this particular essay by Rogers to be "wonderfully, endearingly truthful on the one hand, and on the other hand, somewhat deceptive in what he left out, he was thus perpetuating an image of himself that was only partly accurate." Kirschenbaum was quick to point out: "The moral here is that you probably can't fully trust anything I, or anyone else tells you. Consciously or not, we offer an incomplete and possibly misleading picture."

Kirschenbaum was particularly interested in this incomplete picture because, after writing what he thought was the definitive biography of Rogers' life, he was granted access to the man's personal journals that were chock full of disclosures and secrets that Kirschenbaum, and few others, could have ever imagined. He was so surprised after discovering Rogers' lifelong battles with depression and alcoholism, his sexual confusion, his struggles with being understood, his mental exhaustion, and, yes, his denial of aging, that Kirschenbaum (2008) wrote a new, updated biography exploring these and other issues.

Like Kirschenbaum, many people approaching traditional retirement age, therapists among them, consider the importance of leaving some legacy behind, some indelible footprint that they walked the earth and left an impression behind them long after they were gone. We are not just talking about genetic material, but also the result of some effort that helped make the world a better place, even if in a small way.

Existentialist-oriented therapists, and those who practice what has been called *life review* or *reminiscence therapy* (Butler, 1963; Butler, 1974; Rando, 2000) have well-developed treatment protocols to facilitate the work of articulating a legacy among older clients. The goal is to help people to maintain a consistent sense of self in the face of age-related changes (Molinari, 1999). Much of this is connected to those life activities, past and present, that will be remembered and appreciated in some way. Of course, in our profession, we are especially fortunate in this regard in that our work continues to live and flourish in the minds and hearts of all those we have helped.

SECRETS OF THE OLDER THERAPIST

There are certain secrets of highly active adults, just as more experienced therapists have developed tricks of the trade to function more efficiently. In one study of elderly individuals living in residential facilities, those who remained most active and engaged discovered ways to keep themselves involved in a variety of social activities and physical regimens. In addition, they managed to do so regardless of external factors such as weather, transportation problems, living situation, and resources available (Franke et al., 2013). They offered no excuses for postponing planned activities and they relied consistently on their strengths to compensate for other limitations.

One 71-year-old resident, for instance, suffered from fibromyalgia and yet followed a cardio and weight-lifting regimen every day without fail, even when it meant walking in all kinds of conditions to the local community center. He awakened every morning at 4:45 a.m. and walked to the center, where he spent two to three hours every day keeping himself in the best possible shape. This is the kind of determination and commitment to remain active that best predicts maximum functioning. When asked how he managed to continue this plan, given his chronic disease, he pointed in particular to social support: "I've been going there for years and years and years. And so a lot of the regular people, we know each other. We're friends" (Franke et al., 2013, p. 404).

In the case of senior therapists, they have also developed social networks over time, interpersonal resources that allow them to continue to operate at the highest level, whether in their work or daily life. In addition, as exemplified by Pat Love's experience, a therapist who works with couples, she has learned to become far more efficient and present with her clients. "Even though research, reasoning, supervision, and seasoning have made me smarter, that's not the biggest difference between the sophomore and senior me. A before-and-after video would show a calmer demeanor and more attuned presence—at least that's my experience, and my expectation is clients would say the same."

Pat acknowledged that, out of necessity, she has had to become far more adaptive because of obvious shortcomings. "I no longer have the jet-fueled drive I used to have to make things happen. And I resent the fact that I'm a technology immigrant rather than a native. I think there should be a special word for computer rage when you know your work is in there but can't find it. It's also challenging to avoid the 'meh' response when yet another new theory comes along that I learned three decades ago and was called something else. It's also hard for me to keep my mouth shut about it."

One thing that makes it easier for Pat to continue growing and learning is that she has managed to retain much of her passion and curiosity. "I still very much like what I do. In fact, there is rarely a day that goes by that I am not grateful for meaningful work. I live in gratitude that I have exciting thoughts, delicious ideas, new theories. I still love reading research, creating strategies, and helping people. I appreciate having the skills and knowledge to make others' lives better. I see so many people my age or younger who are bored, apathetic, and depressed because they have no clear purpose in life. My purpose is still clear—even clearer."

LEARNING TO BE FLEXIBLE AND ADAPTIVE TO CHANGES

It is our job as therapists to teach people how to deal with change, whether the result of desired goals or circumstances beyond their control. In the case of older adults, many of these changes are related to some kind of physiological process. Something breaks down or happens to them. Roughly half the people who reach the age of 80 are going to experience some kind of major physical malady, if not a significant disability related to mobility, sensory or cognitive function, or chronic pain. And yet, despite such challenges, some people are able to adjust to the difficulty and maintain a high quality of life satisfaction and enjoyment.

There are two kinds of abilities related to this successful adjustment, both of which are within our purview to teach clients as well as ourselves. The first, *assimilative coping,* involves learning ways to accomplish goals and desired tasks by experimenting with alternative strategies; the second, *accommodative coping,* means altering one's goals (Brandstedter, 1990).

Hill (2005) mentions an example in which, in the first case, if visual loss makes it difficult to read the newspaper, one can use a magnifying glass to assimilate an alternative coping strategy. And if and when that no longer works well, the person could accommodate further by listening to the radio or audio media, or deciding that staying current with news is no longer a priority. In both cases, older people can be taught and encouraged to make the best of their situations instead of remaining focused on the losses. Flexibility appears to be the order of this stage in life, and people desperately need coaching to learn ways to become more accepting of things that can't be changed and to learn to be more open to new possibilities.

Although not exactly "old," more like middle age, a therapist turning 50 reflected on the ways she functioned differently in sessions than when she was younger. Bermann (2009) was asked by a client how her vacation had been and she simply replied it had been fine. But, she felt awkward with the inherent inequality of their relationship and so had naturally deflected the questions, afterward feeling guilty that she had lied when, in fact, her time off had been a major disappointment. "I feel the echo of this in the patient's question, and sometimes it evokes a longing, which the patient may share, for a different kind of connection" (p. 268).

Thinking back to when she was younger, Bermann realized that she was now far less timid than she had been when she first started out. She noted the ways she felt so much more confidence, and willingness to take risks, that she would not have considered earlier in her career. She decided to confront her patient's obvious annoyance at her brisk, rejecting, and dishonest response and instead offered a far more frank answer. She admits she never would have had the courage to do this previously and it provided a breakthrough in their relationship. "I might say that as a result of age, and my practices, I was a bit more able to relax into my discomfort than I had been in the past" (Bermann, 2009, p. 269).

Helen Hudson, a considerably older therapist, described herself as having been born to work with elderly clients. "I was raised by both my grandmother and great-grandmother. As a result, seeing wrinkled faces, mottled skin and watching arthritic great-granny maneuver through the house with her walker was normal for me" (Irving, 2013, p. 28). Growing up with caregivers helped her to develop tremendous compassion and empathy for older people, skills that not only assist her in her work but also facilitate her own adjustment. She's learned along the way some important lessons that may be counterintuitive for those who aren't used to working with this population. The first of which is that it often isn't necessary to spend much time developing rapport and building trust as we might with resistant adolescents: "If they are coming for help, they have a pretty good reason why they need it and usually a stronger sense of time urgency to achieve it" (p. 28). Be that as it may, although we acknowledge this might be true for some of her clients, our experience is that sometimes older clients find the relationships we forge with them to be the main reason why they are there. They crave the intimacy, attention, and responsiveness we offer them that is missing in their lives.

Hudson does make the valid point about the incredible diversity of so-called older clients, citing examples of a 50-year-old who was unexpectedly going through a divorce, the 60-year old who was anxious about life after retirement, the 70-year-old who was struggling with a terminal illness, and the 80-year-old who had trouble with self-care.

MAKING CONNECTIONS, REGARDLESS OF AGE AND STAGE OF LIFE

As in everything else that we do to help people, it is primarily through a relational connection that we help our clients feel understood and develop sufficient trust to accomplish the therapeutic goals that have been negotiated.

In studies that examine factors that are most likely to lead to a solid therapeutic relationship, perceived complementarity seems to be key. Clients who see their therapist as similar in terms of culture, religion, and age are more likely to stick around and be more satisfied with treatment. Rosen, Miller, Nakash, Halpern, and Algeria (2012) found that, in particular, clients who are closer in age to their therapist tend to be much happier with the outcome and view the relationship in more positive terms. This presents some challenges for younger therapists who work with older clients in that the age disparity between participants should be discussed openly in sessions rather than pretending the generational gulf does not exist at all.

JEFFREY: WHAT GOES AROUND, COMES AROUND

I was only 21 years old when I was first hired as a substance abuse therapist; the worst part is that I appeared so much younger than my stated age. Most of my clients were seasoned addicts almost twice my age and I was often not taken seriously because, first of all, I wasn't a recovering addict myself, and second, I looked like I was still in high school. During the ensuing years it felt like I fought an ongoing battle to overcome the handicap of my youth.

When I was a doctoral student, still only 23, I was assigned to teach a counseling course at an extension of my university at Quantico Marine Base. My students were retiring colonels in their 50s who were looking for a career change. (Don't ask me why they wanted to switch from marine officer to a counselor.) Needless to say, I had my hands full and that legacy had followed me most of my life.

Until recently.

Because I have long been aware of the barriers in place when there are great age differences with our clients (or students) now I have an opposite problem. I have little difficulty connecting immediately with "mature" individuals, but notice the wary looks I sometimes get from adolescents in sessions or students in their early adulthood. I can hear them thinking, "How can this old dude possibly understand me and my problems?"

Payback is a bitch.

Two prominent theoreticians in the psychotherapy field, Robert Wubbolding, a reality therapist, and Claudia Black, an addictions specialist, have both discovered wonderful gifts they've enjoyed as a result of their vast experience over many decades of practice—and living. Although each of them subscribes to therapeutic approaches that involve specific techniques and interventions, their success as practitioners is based, in part, on their ability to connect with people. This is possible largely because of their vast life experiences and their willingness to examine deeply their own internal ways of coping with advanced age.

For Wubbolding, he has become far more philosophical and curious. "I realize, and accept," he says, "that we weren't meant to live here permanently. We are all just passing through."

As he approaches the prospect of the end of his life, he wonders what happens next. "Many writers have used metaphorical language, the only kind we have available to us, in an attempt to describe what is next. However, in the last analysis they all say, 'We don't know.' But still at this stage of my life I wonder . . . ."

Because of this uncertainty, Wubbolding feels a much greater imperative to appreciate every moment, to live in the here and now even with an eye toward a tenuous future. It helps that the ideas he was once introduced to as a beginner in his 20s finally begin to make sense in later life. "I learned the concepts but did not *really* understand their depth."

It bothers him a lot to hear someone say that he's growing old gracefully. "I can honestly say I am not growing old gracefully. I am, and I will always, fight it every step of the way. This fight is not a hostile conflict, however. It is a refusal to accept the debilitating characteristics of seasoned citizenry. I hope that more and more senior therapists will remain active and continue to contribute to the profession by teaching, writing, and making their voices heard."

Claudia Black has also noticed—and enjoyed—some of the benefits that have developed through growing older and more experienced. "Compared with my younger years I believe that, if anything, I am more relaxed as a result of confidence in both my skills and trusting the process of therapy. I hold clients more accountable for what they get out of therapy than I think I did in my earlier years."

She has observed that many of the younger, less experienced therapists she has supervised don't often appreciate that sometimes less is better. "As I've grown older I may not work the length of hours, or with the intensity, or be so perfectionistic as I once was. I am less driven, and I think that is good. I no longer feel compelled to read the vast amounts of literature in the field as I once did; I do not do as much prep work ahead of a session as previously. Others may not appreciate that, in fact, what may appear as less may be just as good, if not better."

As older therapists we have an obligation to help other senior people with their issues. These are people who can only be served by others who understand personally the depth of the transition that is being described.

JON: TALKING TO A CLIENT, TALKING TO MYSELF

Rachel, a former client, came to see me yesterday and apologized for not staying in touch after so many years since we had last met. I indicated that I understood and also felt sorry as I know that, during part of this time, I was dealing with my own medical problems and thus was unavailable to work with her, or anyone else.

Rachel began our reunion by catching me up on the trials and tribulations of her life. She was recovering from a stroke and a heart attack. This had led to other calamities, including an aneurism, nerve damage, chronic pain, and multiple back surgeries involving plates and rods. I sat speechless as she described her current difficulties with turning her head and even going up and down stairs. She talked about many of the "kids" who were trying to help her with pain medications and yet who didn't really understand her situation. She had never felt more isolated and dependent, and never felt so misunderstood.

I remembered how much Rachel loved to travel and that she was especially fond of dancing. She and her husband had taken many international trips that had been focused specifically on learning local cultural dances. She was an active and vibrant grandmother who was, up until this time, the primary caregiver for two of her grandchildren. The last time I saw her she was in the process of learning to do Irish dancing like they did in the theater production *Riverdance*.

I shared my appreciation for her losses and the difficulties with her adjustments to the various physical maladies. I could even understand her plaintive cry that she no longer had any reason to live after losing so many of her interests and passions, and her physical ability to enjoy the things that had always given her the most pleasure.

As I listened, I knew that she wasn't saying she was suicidal as much as she was acknowledging all the losses and felt so despondent. I asked her why she had assumed she could no longer engage in the activities she had so loved, even if she couldn't do them the same ways she had in the past. She couldn't lift her grandchildren any more, but that didn't stop her from loving and caring for them. She was no longer spry on her feet, but that didn't mean she couldn't enjoy renewing her love of more modest dances. And just because her mobility was compromised didn't mean she couldn't travel with a wheelchair that would stabilize her back and neck.

Our work together during the ensuing sessions involved brainstorming ways she could continue engaging in those things that had always given her pleasure in the past, but just to do them differently. The interesting thing is that, given that I am the same age as Rachel, I couldn't help but personalize the messages I was sending her way. I used to love to run and now I walk. I used to so enjoy working 12-hour days and now I'm adjusted to half those hours to function at my best. As I was talking to my client, I couldn't help but talk to myself and remember that losses do not really stick until such time that we give up on alternative ways of meeting some of those same needs and desires.

TRICKS OF THE TRADE WORKING WITH OLDER CLIENTS

Therapists who work with older clients face a number of additional challenges that may not be present for their younger clients. The first thing to come to mind is the perceived cognitive deterioration that could lead to reduced capacity for insight or even hearing. But, we make all kinds of adjustments for people, depending on their background, personality, presenting complaints, and other factors. The real problem is that there are very few useful constructs for working with the elderly, and even fewer outcome studies (Hyer, Yeager, & Scott, 2011).

Tailoring treatment to the client is something that all good therapists do; working with older clients presents some unique areas to consider. The first has to do with the ability to communicate via talk therapy.

Seasoned older therapists who have acknowledged and accepted some of their limitations talk openly to their clients about these issues at the onset of treatment. They may begin sessions by mentioning they can't hear as well as they once did and would appreciate it if the client would speak a little louder. They are also inclined to take notes, which may not have been necessary when they were younger. Talking about these adjustments to older clients helps them to feel more comfortable in making clear their own challenges might require certain accommodations.

Adaptations begin with making sure that treatment is offered in a positive and hopeful fashion. Too many services to this population reflect the general pessimism toward older adults. Therapy with this population can be no less successful than with other age groups.

Assistive technology for hearing and vision loss abounds for the elderly, but there are so many other ways to help the aging client. Consultants can be found to make the living space safe and to install bars in the bath and shower area, to remove loose rugs, and to discuss other environmental modifications. Therapists need to be aware of the various technologies available for all aspects of living—from scooters to raised toilet seats to voice-controlled computers.

Autonomy, personal control, independence, and empowerment are variables to consider when working with elderly clients. The elderly want and have earned the greatest respect, and want to be able to keep as much self-control and independence as can safely be allowed. Many have trouble accepting help from caregivers because they want to be known as independent and able to take care of themselves.

Relaxation and meditation are often helpful skills for the older client, as well as the therapist, to learn. Being able to calm oneself and to reduce emotional overreactions to daily frustrations can pay big dividends for reducing fears and stress levels.

Because the elderly have many challenges facing them, therapists often focus slowly on remediation and forget to make happiness, fun, and joy a part of the treatment plan. It is important to discover the pleasant and happily anticipated events and activities in the client's life, and to develop actively ways to increase their frequency.

When working with the "oldest old," it is often useful to expand the definition of who is the client. Given that more than half of all family caregivers of the elderly struggle with their own depression and stress it is important to examine family issues that arise (Hyer et al., 2011). This is not only important for providing support, but also to prevent elder abuse. In one study it was found that the majority of caregivers engage in some form of verbal or even physical abuse when frustration reaches the boiling point (Cooney, Howard, & Lawler, 2006).

This isn't as surprising as it should be considering that, in many cases, family members—without any particular training—are working 24/7 for individuals who have lost the capacity for self-care or informed decision making.

Most professional associations offer specific guidelines for the treatment of older adults, and we cover some of the standards of care and specialized strategies in later chapters. Yet, many of these techniques and practices are geared primarily for symptom remediation rather than focusing on improving the enjoyment, satisfaction, and quality of daily life, regardless of physical limitations. One of the first places to begin this additional focus is by exploring satisfactions that result from wisdom and creativity.

CHAPTER 6
On Wisdom and Creativity

We learn wisdom from failure much more than from success. We often discover what will do, by finding out what will not do; and probably he who never made a mistake never made a discovery.
Samuel Smiles, Scottish philosopher

One of the most influential models of human development that actually covered most of the life span was developed by Erik Erikson and ended with his last stage of Integrity versus Despair. It was only after his wife, Joan, experienced a number of crippling disabilities toward the end of life that she expanded her husband's work and decided to add a ninth stage based on their own increasing difficulties in their 90s coping with the challenges they faced (Erikson & Erikson, 1989). This was hardly a celebration of wisdom and creativity as much as it was a reflection of difficult realities and adjustments. Eventually, if the previous stages were resolved successfully and despair was kept at bay, they believed that *gerotranscendence* may result. This was surmised to be a kind of cosmic communion with the universe, ultimate wisdom that reduces the fear of death and leads to some ultimate engagement as a state of being.

INNOVATION OR IDEALIZATION

What happens to accomplished and successful artists when they reach an age of infirmity? They adapt and soldier on, often developing completely new styles that result in their most heralded masterpieces. This is true for therapists as it is for artists.

It may be well known that Georgia O'Keefe and Grandma Moses created some of their most important works well into their 80s, but so, too, was Michelangelo offered the commission to design St. Peter's Cathedral in his 70s—and that was during a time when the maximum average life span was 20 years younger.

Titan, Picasso, and Matisse also continued remarkable creative productivity as they aged, developing new techniques and inventing new artistic signatures that allowed them to continue working. Claude Monet, one of the founders of impressionism, became enfeebled later in life yet continued to paint his famous water lilies. In fact, he became even more discerning and self-critical as he aged, destroying three-quarters of his canvases that did not meet his standards. So, too, did Renoir have to adapt his technique when arthritis made it difficult for him to hold a brush with his thumb, or Degas whose eyesight failed during later years, and then adjusted accordingly. In each case, these artistic geniuses narrowed their focus during their final periods to continue their creative output in different ways.

So, it turns out that when Albert Einstein claimed that unless one makes a great contribution before the age of 30 he or she would never do so, he was only reflecting his own experience of barren ideas in later life, at least with regard to scientific innovation. Yet even Einstein continued creative work in later life by expanding in other fields of endeavor that allowed him to use his influence for greater good. Representing this kind of change in creative focus, Einstein became more engaged in issues of public policy just as Freud switched his interests from psychotherapy to sociocultural–historical questions of interest, or just as Carl Rogers devoted his later years to applying his theories to world peace and conflict mediation.

Whether old age is truly a time for enlightenment, wisdom, and the final stage of creative innovation, or if such an idea represents an overidealization, the reality is that we don't know very much about this phenomenon on a large scale because the concept is so new. It is certainly the case that extreme images are often presented of the aged, either representing them as debilitated has-beens who've lost all their creative juices, or stating unduly optimistic proclamations of the elderly as having wonderful opportunities to reinvent themselves while minimizing or ignoring the inherent realities of this stage in life. We do know the aging brain is different than its younger version—and that results in qualitatively and quantitatively different output.

These are the facts we mentioned previously that are worth reconsideration when discussing wisdom and creativity: (a) the brain continually evolves, adapts, and reforms itself in light of new experience and learning; (b) contrary to popular belief, new brain cells do develop and proliferate throughout life until the very end; (c) the brain increases its ability to function in a more balanced way, using both hemispheres far more equally; and (d) emotional circuitry and responsiveness become more mature and measured over time (Moody & Sasser, 2015).

LATE BLOOMERS

It is one of the myths of our culture that invention and creativity exist primarily within the domain of the young and spirited. The dominant narratives of innovation tell the stories of visionaries such as Wolfgang Mozart, Marie Curie, Pablo Picasso, and Orson Welles—all child prodigies whose creativity blossomed in their youth. Likewise, the tech wizards such as Steve Jobs, Mark Zuckerberg, and Bill Gates all made revolutionary contributions to the birth of Silicon Valley in their 20s. Our culture is fascinated by these stories of precocious youth, celebrating individuals who showed such early promise.

Yet there appear to be *two* cycles of creativity during the life span, one for young geniuses (such as T. S. Eliot and Herman Melville) and the other for old masters who don't find their stride until well past middle age. This alternative narrative provides so many other examples of creative geniuses who didn't discover their creative spirit until their 50s or 60s. Talk about adaptation to bodily changes with aging! Grandma Moses began her distinguished career as an artist after arthritis forced her to abandon embroidery. Wallace Stevens was an insurance salesman until his 50s when he discovered a latent talent for writing poetry. Ditto with Maya Angelou who wasn't recognized for her writing until her 60s. Some of the most influential political figures of the last century—Golda Meir, Winston Churchill, Nelson Mandela, and Ronald Reagan—were well into their 70s when they served in office. Alfred Hitchcock never achieved excellence as a film director until he was well past 50. Johann Wolfgang von Goethe began writing *Faust* when he was 59, but didn't complete this seminal work until he was 83. Similar trajectories are evident, as well in the lives of Julia Child, Daniel Defoe, and so many others (Box 6-1).

BOX 6-1 INDIVIDUALS WHO WERE EXTRAORDINARILY CREATIVE IN LATER LIFE

Pablo Picasso
Igor Stravinsky
Frank Lloyd Wright
Martha Graham
William Carlos Williams
Willem de Kooning
Robert Frost
Wallace Stevens
Alfred Hitchcock
Daniel Defoe
Mark Twain
Paul Cezanne
Sigmund Freud
Benjamin Franklin
Nelson Mandela
Julia Child
Mother Teresa
Mahatma Gandhi
Grandma Moses
Maya Angelou
Giuseppe Verdi
Charles Darwin
Henry Ford
Bertrand Russell
Frank Lloyd Wright
Coco Chanel

One fascinating story, mentioned by Goldberg (2005) in his book on the neurological changes that take place with aging, describes how Willem de Kooning, the founder of abstract impressionism, became one of the most important artists of the 20th century during his 75-year-long career. He was fueled by creativity, always striving to develop new visions of his art instead of following a familiar and wildly successful pattern. In later life he started to lose his memory to Alzheimer's disease, sometimes unable to recognize his closest friends. Yet, in one sense, forgetting his past helped him to reinvent himself every day as he continued painting with a passionate fury. At age 81 he remarked about his method, "A finished painting is a reminder of what not to do tomorrow." His loss of cognitive functioning with age actually became a gift in that it freed him up to approach each blank canvas with a completely fresh palette.

Kluger (2013) catalogued examples of creative productivity among the elderly, noting historical figures who did some of their innovative work during an age when others have long retired. Frank Lloyd Wright started designing the Guggenheim Museum in New York, perhaps his most famous building, when he was 76 years of age, and didn't complete the project until he was 86. Galileo, who lived during a time when the average life expectancy was about 35, continued publishing scientific papers when he was twice that age. Francisco de Goya completed some of his greatest masterpiece paintings as he approached 80 years of age. Likewise, Pablo Picasso was still active as a painter until 90, just as novelist Herman Wouk completed his last novel after the age of 100. Rather than simply doing the same things over and over, following a template established early in life, each of these individuals remained "nimble, adaptive, even visionary, to invent ideas and solve problems on the fly rather than just responding to the same questions with the same answers again and again" (Kluger, 2013, p. 46).

The field of psychotherapy is replete with examples of influential figures who made their most significant contributions in later life. As mentioned earlier, Freud completely reinvented himself when he hit 60, translating his varied interests in history, anthropology, literature, and archaeology, to move away from psychic internal conflict to study tensions between individual motivation and cultural patterns. Later, he went way out on a limb, delving into theological and religious issues that are often common interests of older individuals. Norbert Weiner, the father of cybernetics (and hence systemic theory), published his classic book on the subject when he was in his 50s. So many others have followed in his footsteps; in fact, many of the visionaries within our field—Virginia Satir, Fritz Perls, Milton Erickson, Alfred Adler, Carl Rogers, Murray Bowen, Carl Whitaker, and so many others—may have developed some of their seminal ideas earlier in their careers, but their major influence was exerted during their years of senior status.

JON: A LIFETIME TO SEE MYSELF MORE CLEARLY

It was sometime during my early 60s that I realized that something strange had happened. I couldn't exactly describe the difference, but people were paying more attention and wanting my input more than usual. I have always been a fairly competent therapist and teacher, but something unexpected began to happen. I had always considered myself a prodigy of youth, but now I was beginning to consider that I might actually be a late bloomer.

I began to see different ways to put ideas together, and I noticed patterns in how people behaved. These patterns were always there, but I never seemed to realize their significance. I felt more confident and poised in meetings and speaking to audiences. I jettisoned my previous wardrobe and started wearing Hawaiian shirts to reflect my new level of comfort and informality.

I used to plan classes or workshops with obsessive care and now I seem to be able to riff on almost any topic with a moment's notice. This isn't because I know so much, but because I trust myself to speak whatever truth comes to mind. I know and accept that I'm good at what I do, and it took most of my lifetime to realize and acknowledge that.

A DIFFERENT KIND OF CREATIVITY IN LATER LIFE

The accumulation of knowledge can be classified as both descriptive and prescriptive. Although the former is about the way things are, the latter is more about the way things could be (Goldberg, 2005). Some of the most visionary talks of all time make this distinction. In one review of the greatest and most influential speeches, Duarte (2010) deconstructed and analyzed their underlying structure and formulae and discovered that they had similar features consistent with presenting predictive knowledge. She focused, in particular, on Abraham Lincoln's "Gettysburg Address," Martin Luther King's "I Have a Dream" speech, and Steve Jobs' introduction of the iPod as each of them, in their own way, led to transformative changes in the larger culture.

The cadence and rhythm of each of these seminal speeches alternated between descriptions of what is or used to be ("Four score and seven years ago our fathers brought forth"), contrasted with what might be possible ("It is for us the living, rather, to be dedicated here to the unfinished work which they who fought here have thus far so nobly advanced"). In Dr. King's "Dream," he similarly contrasted the status quo with a vision of the future when freedom and equality might replace hatred and racism. Likewise, when Steve Jobs described a new world in which it was possible "to carry a thousand songs in your pocket," things would never be the same. Although Jobs may have been a genius rather than a representative of wisdom (given his priorities), his speech illustrated most clearly the power of comparing the past and present with a far more inspirational future.

It turns out there are actually different brain mechanisms involved in each of these sources of knowledge, both housed in the cerebral cortex. According to Goldberg's research (2005), descriptive knowledge resides primarily in the temporal, parietal, and occipital lobes whereas prescriptive, visionary knowledge (also known as *wisdom*) is centered on the frontal lobe. In the evolution of the brain, this is the most recently developed area, one that is far less centered on the self and is more focused on collective, community-centered knowledge.

As hopeful and visionary as it might be to imagine an optimistic future in which anything is possible, if aging teaches us one that it is being realistic. When Erik Erikson first described his last stages of human development, he conceptualized wisdom, as opposed to despair and regret, stemming from the kind of maturity in which it is recognized that, although certain things are no longer feasible, there are still other possibilities within the limited time left. This means wisdom is not just about knowing things, but also includes a realistic assessment of one's own limitations.

WHAT IS WISDOM AND HOW DO YOU KNOW IF YOU'VE GOT IT?

Some of the researchers of developmental changes in later life are uncomfortable with the concept of wisdom as a trait worth defining, much less exploring, because it's a term that has been bandied about for thousands of years. Nevertheless, Korkki (2014) consolidated what is generally understood about the nature of wisdom and its properties among elders, including contributions from ancient philosophers as well as contemporary researchers. It's clear that this label has multiple components rather that captures any single quality (Box 6-2).

No matter the physical restraints and cognitive decline, wisdom is really about being able to make sound decisions and adapt to changing circumstances. This is consistent with what many people associated with this trait highlighted as most significant (Holliday & Chandler, 1986). Certainly it involves an exceptional degree of a deep understanding of things, but this is accompanied by extraordinarily sound judgment related to making decisions in the best interest of all parties concerned. There is, thus, a flavor of selflessness and altruism.

Rosanne Tadsen, a retired school counselor, now works in a counseling center. She has found a renewed vigor and passion for her work in this new stage of life even as she struggles with medical issues related to her advanced age. Her excitement is

BOX 6-2 CHARACTERISTICS OF WISDOM AMONG ELDERS

- Nuanced reflection on accumulative experience
- Sensitivity to subtle differences
- Pattern recognition of quality and quantity of information
- Pragmatic coping skills
- Embracing versus resigned acceptance of reality
- Tolerance for cultural and individual differences
- Self-insight and clarity
- Emotional regulation and equanimity
- Critical awareness of personal history
- Acknowledgment of failures and losses
- Ability to settle for less and accept simplification with relief versus disappointment
- Ability to set goals that are realistic and attainable
- Commitment to continued learning and growth
- Understanding of major priorities
- Compassion and focus on others
- Generativity and generosity toward others
- Facing existential despair with faith and humility
- Reflection on meaning and structure of one's life

contagious. "I have always found people and their struggles and stories to be fascinating. I am even more intrigued since I am now viewing the life span from my own wider lens based on so many decades of experience."

She has learned to value her personal losses and suffering from earlier in life because of the lessons she has learned that have added so much richness and such a deeper understanding of her clients' issues and struggles. She has also accrued the wisdom of being able to apply to herself what she teaches others. "I can quiet my mind and focus on the client in a way that I could not previously. I am more patient and able to uncover important details that I would have missed earlier in my career. However, I am also less patient with people who do not respect my time by not taking counseling seriously or by canceling or rescheduling appointments at the last minute. Part of this impatience is a result, I am certain, of the knowledge that my own time is limited."

Time is indeed much more precious as we age. Older people feel the need to be more selective in what they do and how they do it. Even with the feeling that time is speeding up there is also a desire to slow things down as much as possible. There is often a greater appreciation for enjoying the simplest moments.

THINKING AND PROCESSING DIFFERENTLY

In a review of the research related to how older adults tend to think differently as they age, Jeste and Oswald (2014) described characteristics that are quite consistent with what we often call wisdom. One feature that is especially present in the aged is better emotional regulation. The elderly tend to be much more measured and less reactive to stressful situations, experience fewer negative emotions in general, and their memories are colored by a definite positive bias. No matter what they have suffered or how many difficulties they have faced in life, they are more inclined to demonstrate resilience and what has been called posttraumatic growth.

Older adults show a greater tolerance for uncertainty and ambiguity. They are more inclined to recognize the limits of knowledge, acknowledge multiple perspectives, and show a greater willingness to compromise. In the absence of any verified truth, they are more willing to accept the absence of one correct solution to problems. Their reasoning tends to be more nuanced.

As far as decision making is concerned, it is hardly surprising to learn they are better able to postpone immediate gratification than the young and to look for long-term benefits rather than short-term gains. In addition, they exhibit greater compassion, empathy, and altruism than they did earlier in life. All of this adds

JEFFREY: CRYING WITHOUT SHAME

It's interesting when researchers talk about how better emotional regulation evolves with age because I'm not sure that's my experience in every domain. I know they are referring to equanimity in the face of crises or challenges, since supposedly we have seen it all before—or at least something similar. Although I agree that is probably the case, I have also found that I have become far more emotionally expressive in later life. I cry at the drop of a hat.

In the last week alone I cried trying to tell a story about one of our scholarship girls in Nepal who was accepted to medical school—the first in her village ever to attend higher education. I cried talking to my son about wanting to live long enough for his three-year-old daughter to remember me. I cried watching the film, *Selma,* when the civil rights marchers were beaten almost to death. I am even holding back tears this moment as I recollect these incidents.

I had read somewhere that men do become more emotional as they age, and that has certainly been true for me. But perhaps it is less about physiological changes than it has to do with giving up shame. I cry proudly now rather than hold back tears. It is one of the aspects of aging that I now appreciate and honor the most.

up to individuals who are often more concerned with community welfare than with purely self-centered needs.

Although it is certainly the case that younger people think and act much more quickly than those who are older, one significant quality of wisdom involves a much more shaded, sensitive, and critical exploration of problems and situations. Younger people may have an advantage in much faster cognitive processing, but for older people the challenge is that they must sort through much more information to settle on optimal conclusions. It is a case of the tortoise and the hare, although the tortoise may appear to be moving slowly and steadily because she has so much more life experience and accumulative data to review, but this often lead to better outcomes.

A couple had been in therapy together for almost two years, reporting to their new, older therapist that things had not gone well and that it had mostly been a colossal waste of time. They found it difficult to articulate a single benefit that had resulted from all their investment of time and money.

"Tell me more about that was like," the therapist prompted, not wanting to make the same mistakes.

"Well," the wife answered immediately, "we went week after week mainly to talk about how my husband's abuse—" She stopped for a moment and pointed at him. "—reignited post-traumatic stress from my childhood when my father used to beat me."

"That's not exactly true," the husband jumped in. "We've talked about this before and you know how much I love you. I'd never do anything to hurt you."

The wife nodded, looking over at her husband. "Yeah, yeah, I know. But he just asked me what happened in our previous therapy so I'm telling him."

The wife also explained that their previous therapist had referred her for a psychiatric evaluation for posttraumatic stress disorder and medication, as well as urged her to seek simultaneous individual therapy. All of this seemed to make everything worse over time, not only in their marriage but in her symptoms.

"Tell me about this abuse issue," the therapist asked. He was as different as their previous therapist could be: an older man in his 70s whereas their former therapist was in his mid 30s.

The wife explained that the nature of their conflict together wasn't so much about abuse as feelings of abandonment. Her husband traveled a lot for work, trying hard to support them, but this required him to be out of town a lot. This felt to her like a similar situation growing up with her father gone a lot of the time.

As the therapist listened to their story he was struck by the couple's deep caring for one another. It was clear they were very committed to the relationship and were doing their best to keep things going. He was quite puzzled why their problems had been framed and treated the ways they had been and, perhaps as a function of his age and experience, offered a very different interpretation of their situation.

"First of all," he began slowly, commanding the couple's attention because it was the first time in the session that he was responding to them instead of just asking a few questions, "I agree with the diagnosis of abuse of your former therapist."

"You do?!" they both cried out in shock. "I do indeed. But the only abuse that I see is an abuse of love—meaning, you are both working so hard and will do almost anything for one another, including put up with painful, long separations."

Before the couple could fully process what he said, the therapist added, "And I also agree that you are experiencing posttrauma effects of a difficult childhood, but I'd describe them as posttraumatic *growth* rather than stress."

They both looked puzzled. "Well then, what about when we both get so angry at one another? Or when we—."

The therapist held out his hand. "I'm not saying that you both aren't affected by what happened earlier in your life, or that you don't have some problems with one another. But what I am suggesting is that once you resolve some of these differences between you, and to express your feelings better, you can learn a lot from these experiences, just as you already have."

Whether you agree with the way this case was handled, it illustrates the ways that more experienced—and perhaps wiser and older therapists—can draw on alternative frames of reference and look at presenting problems in a variety of different ways.

WISDOM AS THE PRODUCT OF LIFE EXPERIENCE

The reason why wisdom is most associated with older people and almost never with youth, even in the cases of prodigies or early genius, is that it requires a breadth of experience to be able to recognize patterns that are invisible to those with less accumulated knowledge during a lifetime. Wise individuals are not only smart, but also intuitive in their ability to predict certain events that others would miss. For instance, Brigadier General Bill Mitchell, considered the father of the U.S. Air Force, predicted the Japanese attack in Pearl Harbor within 25 minutes of the actual bombings—and he did so 20 years before anyone else even imagined such a thing was possible. This sort of pattern recognition, putting together data in a meaningful sequence, requires a certain degree of maturity that can only be attained through advanced age.

Goldberg (2005) describes this phenomenon as the "wisdom paradox" in that older people may sacrifice cognitive speed, lose some memory functions, and experience other neurological lapses, yet they are still able to function at optimal levels when it comes to providing critical knowledge to solve problems.

Just as beginning therapists must go through a whole systematic process for assessing client difficulties, sorting through possible assessment possibilities, eliminating options, comparing differential diagnoses, constructing hypotheses, testing their applications, formulating a tentative initial treatment plan—all of which can take several minutes, hours, or even sessions to complete—a more experienced practitioner appears to take multiple, intuitive shortcuts that lead to optimal solutions in seconds, apparently based on very little observable data.

In the language of Jean Piaget, younger people must accommodate new schemas into a limited repertoire of existing concepts whereas older people can accommodate them into a vast number of existing and familiar cognitive templates. Although this can lead to a danger of overgeneralization, in many ways it leads to faster and far more intuitive solutions to problems. Older therapists, for example, may arrive very quickly at a diagnosis or intervention strategy, but they may also overlook novel or unique situations because of overreliance on what is perceived to be familiar. Younger professionals might be more inclined to be cautious and reflective in such scenarios, leading to the obvious conclusion that mutual collaborations across the age span are often ideal.

Wisdom is often described as somewhat effortless decision making when it actually represents an investment of time and energy during a lifetime. There is, thus, an economy of energy expended to compensate for other physiological limitations. As mentioned previously, this helps explain why Nature even allows older people to hang around, even if they can no longer reproduce or contribute to strenuous physical labor. They may not be able to hunt or gather food as effectively as in the past, but they can inform others about the best locations for doing so.

Goldberg (2005) admits that we might think we know what wisdom is when we see it (or think we've attained it), but he quotes Robert Sternberg (1990, p. 3), one of the notable authorities on the subject, that to "understand wisdom fully and correctly probably requires more wisdom than any of us have." Lord Chesterfield echoed that sentiment a century earlier with the observation: "In seeking wisdom thou art wise; in imagining that thou hast attained it—thou art a fool." In that sense, wisdom is a bit different than what we understand as "competence," "expertise," or "genius," because it usually involves making connections between the new and the old, which means vast experience with the past. If genius is an extreme example of talent, then Goldberg (2005) insists wisdom represents an extraordinary degree of expertise. To achieve such a level of competence, a certain amount of maturity and reflective practice are required—conditions that aren't usually possible until later life.

Most of the discussions of wisdom, and its attributes, are discussed in theological literature rather than in the context of human development. There is a distinction between theoretical versus practical wisdom—that is, knowing stuff and knowing how to put the knowledge into action. There is the collective wisdom of a particular group versus that accumulated knowledge of an individual within that group. There is, according to Charles Dickens, "wisdom of the head, and a wisdom of the heart." In all its forms and manifestations, whether in heaven (transcendent) or on Earth, it generally means having good judgment that accrues from life experience. It is about far more than knowing stuff through research, data collection, and observation; it involves deep understanding of essential "truths."

Aristotle defined wisdom as knowledge of essential guiding principles. Plato believed the principle characteristic involved knowing what you don't know, which is especially profound and intriguing as a concept when applied to the practice of therapy. One of my (Jeffrey) early supervisors used to warn me constantly not to worry so much about not understanding what was going on with my clients, but rather to be concerned during those times when I thought I knew what was really happening. He believed that a certain modesty was important to achieve excellence, and this contrasted considerably with others I had known in group supervision conferences who were continually spouting their certainty about my cases, identifying exact diagnoses and recommended treatments, although they had never met my clients and were relying on 10-minute summaries of their experiences.

McKee and Barber (1999) attempted to define wisdom, not in terms of what is known, but rather *how* this knowledge is known. They propose that wisdom primarily involves seeing through illusions that would be obscured or hidden from others. Furthermore, such an ability comes mostly from suffering through illusions, learning from prior failures, and reaching an advanced state of enlightenment. Confucius noted that wisdom can be learned by three sources: "First, by reflection, which is noblest; second, by imitation, which is easiest; and third by experience, which is the bitterest."

We have found in our own research (Kottler & Carlson, 2002, 2009) that extraordinary practitioners have not only attained an extraordinary degree of creative innovation in their work, but also they are also quite forgiving of their mistakes and misjudgments. In the words of two contributors to our studies, Frank Pittman and Cloe Madanes, it is only possible to do exceptional work if one is willing to take risks and experiment with novel solutions to problems.

One of the benefits of living longer and accumulating experience is there is at least the potential to develop a more robust, comprehensive perspective—a sense of wholeness that younger practitioners might miss. This development of greater clarity and wisdom results from a lifetime of facing difficult truths in sessions. Hedda Bolgar, still practicing therapy until her death at 102, summarized this point quite well: "I live by one idea now, which is that in analysis we don't try to avoid things, we don't try to hide things. We are committed to uncovering things and dealing with it" (Bolgar, 2006).

One of the changes that is often reported by older therapists is that they may be less certain of absolute truth, less reliant on supposed accurate diagnosis, and more accepting of complexities and uncertainties. Perhaps Benjamin Franklin said it best that "the doorstep to the temple of wisdom is a knowledge of our own ignorance." Yet such awareness of fallibility is hardly enough. Early 20th-century artist and writer Elbert Hubbard admitted that "every man is a damn fool for at least five minutes every day [but that] wisdom consists in not exceeding the limit." There are so many other great thinkers and philosophers who echo the same idea in their own words. We mention Bertrand Russell as one additional example that we have found especially insightful, and a guiding principle for our own ongoing development as therapists and teachers: "The whole problem with the world is that fools and fanatics are always so certain of themselves, but wiser people so full of doubts."

Throughout most of our careers, we have been both surprised and unnerved by the arrogance of some colleagues who speak with such authority and self-assurance about what they claim to know and understand. We have sat in case conferences and supervision sessions and listened to identified experts talk with perfect confidence about the diagnoses they bestow on clients, as well as the best treatment protocol, always followed by a casual but arrogant statement regarding "this is what research supports." We have sat on panels with colleagues who claim they have cornered the market on truth and anyone who disagrees with them is misguided or stupid.

OLDER PEOPLE DO KNOW LOTS OF STUFF

As we have emphasized, there is a certain amount of knowledge, wisdom, and insight that are accrued by the elderly as a function of their life experiences. They have lived long enough to have encountered many of the challenges faced in everyday existence and they have also learned how to let certain things go that they can't possibly control. They might realize, for instance, that it is futile to try to change other people—a strategy which younger people are often oblivious. A few other things that older people may have learned to let go of include the following (Brenoff, 2014):

1. *Grudges eat away at your soul.* There is the old adage from 12-step programs that the only thing worse than remaining in an ongoing conflict with someone is allow that person to live, rent-free, in your head. The most successful among us have figured out the power of forgiveness, of letting go of resentments toward those who have done you wrong. We are not saying this means opening yourself up to more abuse, but rather that it is best to let go of stuff from the past that continues to fester.
2. *It really isn't about winning, but how you play the game.* There are good reasons why young people are obsessed with competition, status, and achievement. After all, they are programmed evolutionarily to obtain the best position and resources possible to increase the probability that their offspring will have the best opportunities for survival and advancement in the community. For older people it is often far less important to show dominance and power, to win every argument, to be seen as right. Usually what's at stake is relatively,

insignificant and older people have learned to preserve their energy to fight battles that really matter.

3. *It isn't those with the most stuff, or even the most friends, who are fortunate, but rather those who are determined enough to enjoy a few deep, meaningful relationships with loved ones.* Sure, financial stability and comfort are important to a certain degree, but beyond a moderate level, expending effort to accumulate wealth and status is a waste of energy that could be better invested in friendships, family, and creative interests. A corollary to this insight is also knowing that you can't make everyone like you, no matter how much you try. Another variation of this theme, once observed by Alfred Adler, is that "the only normal people are the ones you don't know very well." A deeper truth, learned from life experience, is that everyone has triumphs and joys, as well as sorrows and imperfections.

Robert Stoller (1992) sought to record all the wisdom and advice he had accumulated during his half century of devotion to the practice of therapy. He made a list of insights he considered most important, one of which was somewhat surprising and against the grain of conventional wisdom—but then he admits that one of the privileges of age is that one is allowed to be more opinionated, or at least express one's opinions more forcefully. Although he practiced as a psychoanalyst, confronting distortions of reality and defense mechanisms as his job, he acknowledged that denial could be wonderful thing. It is a kind of "honorable dishonesty" that allowed him to pretend that he truly had the freedom to do whatever he wanted. He recognized that reality would eventually end his "benign game," but hopefully not until he was forced to confront truth when denial became a burden. Ironically, Stoller was only 66 when he wrote down his thoughts, believing he had many years left to complete unfinished business; he was killed in a car accident soon thereafter.

THE REINVENTION OF SELF

Aging is, in part, about reinvention. It is about renegotiating goals and aspirations that are more congruent with resources and skills available. The traditional model for the last 75 years or so since the Industrial Age was in full swing involved joining an organization or company, working until retirement, and then spending the so-called "golden years" puttering in the garden or taking care of grandchildren. Although this is still relatively commonplace, it is far more likely that most older people are choosing new "careers" and interests after they are granted discretionary time to pursue them. One role of therapists is to help clients contemplate new responsibilities and possibilities for the future—in some cases, options that had never been considered before.

Isabelle Bick, an 81-year-old therapist, sees the greatest single impediment to the development of wisdom in people her age is the self-defeating belief that "I can't stand who I am now because I'm not who I used to be" (Korkki, 2014). Instead of whining and complaining about the way things used to be, wise elders have learned to embrace the realities, and even the limitations, of what is no longer within reach, and instead focus on what is within their capabilities still to strive for excellence and feelings of productivity. This can—and should be—a major focus of what we do in sessions with older clients, helping them to assess realistically what they can and can't do, honoring and holding the sadness and sense of loss over what is no longer possible, but also reassessing new and different priorities that can lead them to feel fulfilled. This is extremely challenging to accomplish, which is why true wisdom is so difficult to attain.

RENEWAL OF CREATIVITY

One way that wisdom is often conceived is in terms of questioning the status quo, or at least knowing which questions to ask to arrive at a solution to a problem. "You can tell whether a man is clever by his answers," writes Egyptian Nobel Laureate for literature, Naguib Mahfouz, but "you can tell whether a man is wise by his questions." Wise elders are not only those who hold knowledge, but also those who are able to ask questions that others may not consider. This is certainly the case with regard to what we do in therapy. And it is also true with respect to questioning our own professional roles and engagement as we evolve and learn over time.

Although it used to be the case that old age meant retirement and disengagement from previous activities, more than ever before people are choosing to postpone retirement, and not just for economic reasons, but because they feel they still have much to offer. In one representative study it was found that three-quarters of Baby Boomers did expect to retire when they hit age 64; they planned to begin a new career focused on a longstanding interest (Wright, 2006). In some cases, this might involve volunteer work, but in many instances it could mean a whole new professional enterprise.

As we've noted before, although some intellectual and cognitive functions are compromised with aging, the brain compensates in other ways that have been found actually to improve creative output and problem solving. Functions are reorganized in the brain. Multitasking may become more challenging, but that doesn't change the ability to focus, single-mindedly, on a particular task and produce remarkably creative outcomes based on a breadth of life experience

In a review of things that highly creative people do differently than others it shouldn't be all that surprising that older professionals have greater potential to excel in the domain because of diverse life experiences and "messier" minds—meaning, they are more complex (Gregoire, 2014). Based on this review of research in the field the following factors seem to be most prevalent:

1. *Daydreaming.* A wandering mind may have gotten us in trouble in elementary school, but it turns out that "undisciplined" thoughts can often lead to creative incubation, new insights, and novel connections between disparate elements. Perhaps this is why it's not as unusual as we might imagine that elders are often responsible for breakthroughs and innovations.
2. *Making careful observations.* As therapists we have been particularly trained and forged into the most scrupulous observers of human phenomena. What we do for a living, what we have always done since we entered the profession, is listen and watch people very, very carefully, and make connections between what we have observed and other things that we have observed and experienced. There is nobody else around who is more analytic, more rigorous, and systematic in making sense of the incomprehensible and explaining mysteries that have previously been inscrutable. We see possibilities where others see only limitations. We look deeply into the issues and phenomena that others most avoid. And as we age, we only get better at this ability, refining our skills and becoming even more efficient in seeing through the murky fog that keeps others from reaching their greater potential.
3. *Seeking the silver lining.* All the new advancements in positive psychology and posttraumatic growth point to the benefits of turning suffering, failure, and disappointment into opportunities for learning. In a previous study (Kottler & Carlson, 2002), we interviewed a few dozen of the most prominent elders in our field about their most significant failures and disappointments in therapeutic work. This included theorists such as Albert Ellis, William Glasser, Peggy Papp, and others, many of whom were approaching the end of their life. In looking back on their distinguished careers, they often pointed to their failures as the seminal events that helped them develop breakthroughs in their thinking. It would appear that extraordinarily creative individuals are able to embrace, rather than deny, their mistakes and to use them as data to develop new ideas.

   The older we get, (potentially) the more accepting we can be in coming to terms with our lapses and disappointments. It is easier to shrug them off, or better yet, find their silver linings, when our well-being and confidence will not be shattered as a result. Younger therapists have so much at stake as they begin their careers. Each and every error of judgment and miscalculation—and there are so many—can spin the therapist into a crisis of doubt. But, when we've heard and seen most things before, or at least *think* we have, it makes it easier (in some ways) to take things in stride when they don't go the way we expect. And it is precisely when things don't proceed along expected lines that creative breakthroughs actually most often take place.

Relational–cultural theorist Judy Jordan described how a client once challenged her by asking if there was actual love in their relationship (Kottler & Carlson, 2009). Although initially caught off guard and inclined to deflect the uncomfortable question, eventually Jordan came to terms with a much clearer (and creative) vision of what therapeutic relationships could be when framed in a more genuine and egalitarian way. This is not unlike what Carl Rogers realized in his most stunning creative breakthroughs—that he tended to fail his clients when he put up the most barriers and followed the prescriptions of the time. He was able to abandon what had been foisted upon him by supervisors and colleagues only after he could find his own unique voice, which led him in a very different direction.

4. *Seeking intrinsic motivation.* Creativity is most often driven by passion and desire to make sense of things or to answer a question that has personal resonance. Only very rarely does a breakthrough pay off with some extrinsic reward such as money or fame. Far more often, the benefit is personal satisfaction. So many of our most creative geniuses never knew in their lifetime that anyone appreciated their work. Artists Vincent Van Gogh and Johannes Vermeer, composer Franz Schubert, and poet William Blake all died relatively unknown, and often in poverty. They couldn't support themselves or their families very well but they lived to fulfill their creative spirits.

   Older therapists have much more opportunity, as a function of their standing, to pursue interests and passions that may have been ignored earlier in life. Such creativity can be expressed through any number of endeavors, whether cooking, gardening, pursuing photography, or writing. One of the privileges of being older is the chance to explore new subjects or activities for which there had never been time before.
5. *Taking risks.* This is one of the domains of creativity that older people might be most likely to avoid, but it is considered so critical for innovation and advancement. Risking-taking and adventure-seeking are far more often associated with youth. But, in the terms that we are thinking, we mean more like remaining open to new experiences. This can be challenging for older professionals who may believe they've seen it all before and know most of what there is to know. It is the beginner's mind that questions and challenges everything: Why do we have to do it this way just because that has always been the case?

This is the primary downfall of so-called experts and veterans, believing they have already discovered the best and most efficient way to get things done. Complacency and laziness infect the spirit. We do what is easiest and most familiar rather than challenging ourselves to continue experimenting and taking risks. It is more rare than we'd like to admit that older therapists are willing to abandon what they think they already know and delve into completely new areas.

Among all the features of creativity that we've mentioned, this is the area in which older therapists are most likely to fall short—*way* short. How often do people in their 60s or 80s quit their job and start over, or abandon their favored therapeutic approach in lieu of something new they've discovered? The truth of the matter is, this doesn't happen that often, although there are noted exceptions. We've worked with a number of students who haven't *begun* their entrance into the profession until age 60 or 70!

The key is to keep asking difficult questions, keep challenging what we do and the way we do it. There have always been outliers who, in their ripe old age, still enjoy sparking debate or chaos. The French psychoanalyst Jacques Lacan was famous for his rebellious outbursts, questioning why we even have a 50-minute hour as standard treatment. He reasoned that we do this only for our own scheduling convenience even though some clients need only 10 minutes for a session when they are playing games or hiding and others need a few hours when they are in crisis. Albert Ellis, as well, reckoned that he and his clients could be far more efficient and focused in 25-minute sessions rather than the usual hour. Eventually, systematic research studies are carried out to determine the efficacy of any change or new development in the field, but it all begins with asking questions that challenges the way things are.

One of our friends and colleagues, Bradford Keeney, took the risk to abandon much of what he learned and practiced as a family therapy theorist and embraced his role as a shaman and "trickster" (Kottler, Carlson, & Keeney, 2004). He wondered why our relatively young field of only 100 years would abandon or ignore the wisdom of indigenous healing practices that have been in operation for tens of thousands of years. Talk to any self-respecting shaman in the Kalahari of Africa, Outback of Australia, or tribal group in North America and they find it hilarious that we expect to change anyone by having conversations with them in a sheltered room. Within most indigenous traditions, healing takes place in the community and usually involves shaking, dance, music, rituals, spiritual transcendence, trials, and tasks, but almost never any talk. In fact, when describing what we do in psychotherapy to one Bushman shaman in Namibia, he looked at us and fell over laughing, asking us if we'd ever helped anyone just talking to them. You have to admit that's a pretty good question.

It is a practical reality that anyone who ventures into the realm of creativity, and stands by his or her findings, is taking tremendous risks with reputation and standing in the community. In that sense, elders have far more to lose and may be far more unwilling to risk all they have gained.

There are many other factors related to creativity that are also frequently mentioned—making time for solitude, adapting a work schedule that best fits one's individual preferences, thinking way outside the usual boxes that hold the status quo. In all their forms and manifestations, older people benefit in a number of ways as a result of discovering new forms of creative expression (Cohen, 2006):

1. *Psychological mastery and sense of control.* Being actively involved in some creative interest provides a sense of empowerment.
2. *Maintenance and improvement of physical health.* The sense of control also produces increased immunity accompanied by bursts of positive emotional energy.
3. *Social engagement.* Creative activities often provide increased opportunity for shared experiences. Whether participating in pottery classes, a choral group, or any artistic endeavor, social relationships reduce stress and, even, blood pressure.
4. *Brain plasticity.* There is a documented phenomenon of aging that, at midlife and beyond, there is increased bilateral brain development and functioning. The brain becomes more flexible in integrating tasks that had been limited previously to one hemisphere or the other. Creative activities appear to be especially well-suited to optimizing simultaneous brain stimulation.

Cohen's (2005, 2006) research, as well as other studies (Hanna, 2013; Patterson & Perlstein, 2011; Tsai, 2013), consistently support the notion that, rather than losing brain function irreversibly as we age, there are also opportunities actually to adapt to the changes by accessing different resources. The combination of physical conditioning and creative engagement appears to optimize the potential actually to grow new neuronal dendrites and synapses. As we discussed earlier, the really amazing part is the way the brain learns to reorganize itself to compensate for changes that have taken place.

Even for those older therapists who decide to retire, or at least reduce significantly their active treatment with clients, there are so many ways to use the accumulated wisdom and skills to make a creative impact. Fieldsteel (2011), for example, accepted that it might not be in the best interests of her clients for her to continue practicing, given her age, but she still found many ways to remain professionally active through writing, teaching, and supervising. In fact, she found herself rejuvenated after discovering new ways to make a difference, relying on a metaphor she created: "I have been delighted and intrigued by the artists now working in the area of found art. Using old and sometimes discarded materials, they create new, exciting images and change our view of the world and its possibilities" (p. 16).

The American Association of Retired Persons publishes newsletters each month enthusiastically proclaiming "100 Benefits of Being Retired" or "50 Reasons to Love Being over 50." These are as much exaggerations and lies as the statement that older people are all sages with a fountain of knowledge for which everyone is begging. More often than not, they (we) are treated as obsolete relics of the past whose supposed wisdom is worthless in this new technological world. We next consider some of the other myths and misconceptions associated with growing old.

PART III

Aging Clients

CHAPTER 7
Myths and Misconceptions of What It's Like to Be Old

If growing up means it would be beneath my dignity to climb a tree, I'll never grow up, never grow up, never grow up! Not me!

J. M. Barrie, *Peter Pan*

There is perhaps no more stressful job in the world than serving as President of the United States. The hours are insane. The responsibility of the free world rests on one's shoulders. Life-and-death decisions are just a normal part of the job. No matter what you do, or don't do, roughly half the citizens and most journalists will become rabid, ungrateful critics. You live in a bubble with almost no privacy. And despite lofty goals and grand expectations, it is probable that disappointments are the order of the day. Indeed, there are frequent comments made about sitting presidents that their hair turns prematurely gray within the first few years in office and they have noticeably aged, far more than one would expect, upon leaving the White House.

So, then, it comes as quite a shock to discover that presidents actually have a *greater* than normal life expectancy, surviving five years longer than the population at large (Olshansky, 2011). Even going back to the first eight chief executives—Washington, Adams, Jefferson, Madison, (J. Q.) Adams, Jackson, Van Buren, and Harrison—each lived an average of 80 years when the normal life expectancy of the time was half that! Our most recent presidents have kept this record alive, far exceeding what would be expected. Gerald Ford, Ronald Reagan, Herbert Hoover, George Herbert Bush, and Jimmy Carter lived to be older than 90.

Certainly high-level political leaders would have access to the best possible medical care, and also enjoy the top level of economic prosperity, but that doesn't fully explain the phenomenon. It's also the case in other fields that those at the top of the food chain live longer. For instance, actors who win academy awards live almost five years longer than their peers, just as Nobel Prize winners also outlast others within their field (Szalavitz, 2011). It would seem, then, that stress effects are moderated by attaining some degree of stature within society, regardless of the domain. As we know long ago from the classic "executive monkey" studies, ulcers developed in subjects, not from being shocked, but from not having any control whatsoever over one's situation.

This is a pretty compelling example of why it is so important for us to help empower our older clients, to help them to feel a sense of control over at least some aspects of their life. And it also makes a compelling argument for us to help people to challenge some of the prevailing myths about what it means to be old.

PREVALENT MYTHS ABOUT AGING

Myths are generally based on a lack of accurate knowledge. Over time, they become enshrined as collective beliefs and validated social values. They are also continually confirmed and rarely questioned. Based on a review of the literature, and a study of public perceptions of older people, several stereotypes appear to be most prevalent, at least in Western cultures (Lyons, 2009; Thornton, 2002). These include universal beliefs that older people (a) are disabled, ill, or incapacitated; (b) lack energy and vitality; (c) live in the past because their current days are boring and without much satisfaction and meaning; (d) feel lonely, depressed, and isolated; (e) are generally unhappy and dissatisfied; (f) complain about the way things are because they long for the good ole days; (g) have failing memories and are prone to senility, and (h) are unable to learn because they are too set in their ways.

Other common misconceptions include the belief that most older adults live in nursing homes and cannot get around by themselves; they do little more than sit around and watch television. It is also believed that if older people are able to continue working, it is at a significantly lower level of productivity and efficiency. It is assumed they miss a lot of work days because of illnesses, chronic diseases, and physical disabilities. Furthermore, it is believed they lack any interest in sex, sleep constantly—or not at all—and they are obsessed with death and dying.

One of the most prevailing myths of all is that older people essentially lose their minds. Although it is certainly true that so-called "crystallized intelligence" and cognitive processing speeds do tend to peak during one's 20s, we've mentioned previously how different abilities actually ripen at different ages and stages of life. For instance, although recollection of faces and manipulation of numbers tend to peak at age 30, the ability to read people's moods accurately improves with age and experience. The older brain may indeed operate at a slower rate not only because of decreased functioning in some areas, but also because there is a much larger inventory of data to review. Yet, it is also the case that the eventual conclusions and decisions are more accurate and often produce higher quality results.

Many of the older people with whom we spoke were actually amazed that old age is so different and so much better than they expected (and had been taught to expect). Many indicate they have been waiting for the bottom to fall out and for the advertised lifestyle of "all things bad" to happen. One client disclosed in a session, "It is certainly different than I thought it would be, but it ain't all that bad." She and her husband had been quite busy raising their grandson and were looking forward to their daughter's twins that were due in a couple of months. "We never thought we would have the opportunity, let alone energy, to be parents again, but that is what happened and we seem up to the task. If the truth be told, we seem to have a lot more energy than our daughter and son-in-law. It is as if we have become young again—not exactly the fountain of youth, but similar!"

Of course there are also some positive beliefs associated with aging, often seeing older people as warm, wise, patriotic, knowledgeable, experienced, sincere, cute, good-natured, dependable, religious, and serene, but there are far more negative perceptions. As we have said before, they are often labeled with descriptions as incompetent, shrewd, selfish, stubborn, grumpy, boring, close-minded, bitter, forgetful, depressed, suspicious, intolerant, grouchy, pessimistic, greedy, sick, enfeebled, weak, frail, impaired, dependent, wrinkled, ugly, asexual, conservative, sad, lonely, and isolated.

These perceptions are shaped by a number of factors related to gender, culture, socioeconomic background, geographic location, life experience, level of contact with older people, and especially the age of the person who is asked. Not surprisingly, younger people have more negative views of aging than those who are older, but, surprisingly, those who are middle-aged have the most negative views of all.

Pat Love, an authority on love relationships, has been most frustrated in her own aging journey by the prejudices and myths perpetuated by those her own age. "Perhaps the biggest misunderstanding about this stage of life is the ageism that comes with it." She cites a number of studies that report how older people are often responsible for reinforcing the myths that exist about how they are supposed to behave. This internalized ageism can be crippling. Love remembers the first few times people would say to her, "At your age . . . " and she thought this might be some mistake or misunderstanding. "Over time this attitude can creep into your psyche like a thief in the night and steal your motivation, ambition, and courage to try new ventures."

Love laments that most people don't seem to understand that, regardless of how you look on the outside, you basically feel the same way you always did on the inside. "Even though we look older, our essence is timeless. We live, love, and feel simply like ourselves. The spirit is still willing even though the flesh might be more wrinkled and weak."

Clients—and their families—often bring many of the misconceptions and attitudes about aging into sessions, many of which often influence and even determine their choices and behavior. These can include internalized beliefs that emphasize their sense of helplessness, a situation that, unfortunately, is only reinforced by our culture. In addition, some therapists may implicitly subscribe to them as well without conscious awareness, accepting very limited goals for what can be accomplished in sessions because of a sense of futility.

MYTHS THAT THERAPISTS MIGHT BELIEVE

One of the major impediments to helping elderly clients includes the ways that therapists and other health professionals are "bewitched by the discourses" surrounding what it means to be old, that such cases are hopeless and that prognoses are, at best, only "guarded" and significant improvement is unlikely. Often these negative biases can be counteracted by something as simple as remembering to ask, "What are some of the things that you are perfectly capable of doing that your family doesn't realize or has forgotten?" (Milton & Hansen, 2010). We are talking about looking for exceptions to the difficulties presented, accessing strengths and resources, separating the person from the problem, and focusing on hope and possibilities rather than limitations—all standard brief and narrative therapy protocols (de Shazer, 1985; O'Hanlon, 1993; White, 2000).

JON: THE COW WAS IN LABOR

I spent several years working in a nursing home facility and always left feeling so much better than when I arrived. I would talk to one resident while another would patiently wait for her turn. It didn't seem to matter what we talked about, just that the residents felt heard and understood. Their tired eyes would twinkle as they felt my concern, caring, and interest. It was during this time that I learned just how little the content of sessions mattered.

One day I was met at the door by a desperate woman by the name of Sarah who began screaming, "Doctor, doctor, we need you! Come with me right away!" She took my hand and began to pull and guide me down the hall and into her room where she stopped and pointed to some invisible animal she imagined residing in her room.

"Look," she said, "the cow looks like it's having trouble with the birth. The calf is stuck! You gotta help!"

I was taken aback at first, unsure what was going on. Then, I smiled gently and told Sarah I was not that kind of doctor.

"Oh, well maybe we can just sit here and talk?"

I stayed with her for a half hour and she was surprisingly cogent, telling me about her various grandchildren and great-grandchildren. Although they rarely visited her, and she couldn't remember all their names, she had a remarkable recollection of their ages and favorite activities. I was so enjoying the conversation that I would have stayed longer if I hadn't heard someone moaning and screaming down the hall. One of the staff members asked if I could find out what was wrong and help calm the person down.

I entered the woman's room to find her in bed thrashing around and screaming hysterically. When I asked her what was wrong, just as the staff member had done a few minutes earlier, she just redoubled her moaning. I wasn't sure what else to do except wait patiently for her to settle down. During one pause when she was gathering her breath for another round of wailing, I gently touched her forearm and said in the softest voice, "Is there anything I can do to help you right now?"

Much to my surprise, the woman stopped the impending scream with an expulsion of breath. She looked at me with a shy smile and seemed to hesitate.

"Go on," I encouraged her, "tell me what I can do to help."

"Well, you could get in bed with me. That would make me feel a little better."

I smiled back at her. "Is there anything *else* I can do that would help?"

She started laughing as if we shared this fabulous joke. And that was it. She seemed to regain her composure. I really have no idea why she stopped screaming except that perhaps she wanted some attention. But then, I'm never really that surprised to find that so often what clients need most, and older people in particular, is a feeling of connection.

Not surprisingly, many therapists subscribe to myths about aging as well. Kraus (2012) described how he felt initial reluctance to work with older clients after securing a job in a nursing home facility. He figured they were too cognitively compromised and emotionally restricted to benefit from therapy. And why bother at all because they were so close to death anyway? "I was overwhelmed with confusion, uncertain of my effectiveness, and scared I might be practicing outside my area of competence." Indeed he was!

As mentioned, this is not an unusual predicament considering that so few of us ever have received training in working with the elderly. And the situation is further complicated by some of our own misguided beliefs. After more than a decade adapting to his new specialty, Kraus eventually came to realize what a gift he had received from his elderly clients, how he was learning as much from them as they were learning from him. He found what helped him the most was not so much augmented skills as letting go of some of his misguided assumptions that were getting in the way of being helpful.

Myth number one: It's a waste of time to help older people find meaning in their life because they have so little time left to appreciate and use any gains. On the contrary, it is an even *more* significant achievement to assist an older person in the search for spiritual and psychological peace toward the end of life. Such individuals are not only perfectly capable of participating in such a therapeutic path, but also they are highly motivated to do so. Kraus considers this his most profound professional revelation, one that opened up all kinds of new possibilities for his work with this population.

Myth number two: The problems that older people confront are so entrenched and longstanding it is futile to try and put a dent in them. Everyone knows they are so rigid and inflexible in their beliefs and habits, they are too old to change. You can't teach an old dog new tricks and all that.

There is a myth, or at least a belief, among many therapists, as well as the population at large, that the prognosis for helping elderly clients improve their life is guarded at best. Even more disturbing is the notion that it probably isn't even worth the effort because the changes would be so negligible in light of the severity of various intractable, chronic symptoms. Furthermore, older people are just too damn stubborn to change anyway.

JEFFREY: IMPATIENCE IN ACTION

True confession: In between writing myth one and myth two, I took a break to visit my favorite coffee shop. This is a place for the most insanely discerning palate, coffee snobs totally out of control. They feature exotic blends offered in a setting that resembles a mad scientist's laboratory with fermenting beakers of slow-brewed extract. There was a pair of oldsters in front of me in line and it seemed to take forever for them to settle on their order. Meanwhile, the line was getting longer and the rest of us were becoming impatient. Both of the gentlemen seemed to be hard of hearing and confused by all the choices being described. Then, once they made a decision, they stood there counting change as if they'd never encountered such coins before.

I was seething inside as I waited. I had important stuff to do. Why didn't these old people (actually just a few years older than me) get the hell out of the way? Why were they taking so damn long?

I stopped and took a deep breath, realizing they were in absolutely no hurry because the pace of their lives is so different from mine. And If I intend to become more effective in my work with older clients, I'd better examine more honestly the source of my own impatience.

Myth number three: Old age represents a time of loss and adaptation to deteriorating cognitive and physical functioning. Although this may be strictly true, it is mythical in the sense of how distorted a picture it presents. Kraus likes to ask therapists he's training what they view as the essential signs of aging. Perhaps you'd answer by mentioning things like gray hair, stooped posture, chronic illness, and forgetful memory. But then he offers his primary attributes of old age: wisdom, confidence, character, and strength!

In other words, although aging might be frequently framed in terms of loss of functioning, friends, opportunities, and so on, older adults have a lot less to prove to themselves and others. Ambition and drive for the future have been moderated by a much greater appreciation for enjoying and making the most of the present. What's the rush for Jeffrey to get through the coffee line if the stated purpose of being there is to enjoy and make the most of the recreational break, especially when anticipation is half the pleasure?

WHAT IS AN OLDER THERAPIST "SUPPOSED" TO DO?

In Chapter 3 we discussed some of the advantages and special challenges of older or senior practitioners. Some of these difficulties may relate less to one's age and circumstances than from the particular attitudes, beliefs, and conceptions we hold about what is expected and "age appropriate." Of course this parallels exactly what we attempt to explore with our clients when they also subscribe to ideas that are quite self-limiting.

Social worker Mark Hicks tried retirement at age 65 because he thought that's what he was supposed to do when he hit that magic age. But, he was bored to death. So he upgraded his trifocals and hearing aids (although he couldn't do much for his short-term memory) and resumed work. He learned to make other adaptations, such as to stop asking clients, "Do you remember when . . . ?" Having been born in 1937, hardly anyone still remembers what seems so fresh to him. He recognizes that his clients' frames of reference are now quite different from his own, challenging him to get outside of himself more than ever before. "It helps to remember that I am there to let therapy happen and not force it into place. I have to admit, there are times when I am inclined simply to meet therapeutic challenges with a bigger hammer. But truly understanding their cohort context often helps me to get rid of the hammer altogether" (Hicks, 2012).

In a study of psychiatrists older than 65 who were still in active practice, it was found they were better than younger therapists at metabolizing accumulative stress and adverse effects of continuous exposure to clients' emotional problems and drama (Weiner, 1990). There's that old joke about the young therapist and the elderly therapist meeting in the elevator at the end of the day. The beginner was exhausted, disheveled, and completely out of sorts after an eventful series of sessions whereas the oldster was immaculate in appearance and fresh as ever. "How do you manage to remain so energetic and fresh after listening to your clients all day?" the beginner asked his colleague.

"Who listens?" he answered with a shrug, straightened his bowtie, and skipped out of the elevator whistling to himself.

This is, of course, just a myth. According to Weiner's (1990) series of interviews, although they were conducted many years ago, the older psychiatrists reported tremendous satisfaction and competence in their work—more than ever. And contrary to the previous joke, this was *not* because they maintained energy by disengaging from clients. In fact, most of them struggled with diminished energy, memory lapses, and limitations adapting to contemporary trends and new technologies. Most of them had some type of physical ailment ranging from hearing or vision loss to diabetes, chronic pain, or coronary disease, but nevertheless many said they had adapted fairly well to these limitations and found ways to operate more efficiently in many ways. Of course, like all self-report studies we don't know what their clients would say. Most of the psychiatrists rather honest and clear about their aging effects and so reduced their caseloads and selected less challenging cases.

The elderly psychiatrists noted several other differences in the ways they functioned. For instance, they noticed much less intense countertransference reactions, especially those related to erotic feelings, which would not be surprising among those with reduced libido. They learned to stay within their comfort zone rather than taking on novel cases that might be more than they could handle. In other words, they were more aware of their limitations and willing to stay within them. Finally, they were doing therapy because they loved this work. It was not a job or chore. More and more we hear older therapists describing how they have a perfect vocation.

The older therapists noticed they were more personal and authentic in their sessions than they had been earlier in their careers. They felt they were more hopeful and optimistic about outcomes (possibly because they took on less complex and challenging cases). And they actually seemed to enjoy their work as much as ever before. In the words of one respondent: "There are no books, plays, or movies as interesting as the patients I see each day" (Weiner, 1990, p. 41).

Ann Vernon, a counselor educator for many years, had recently retired and moved into a retirement community, and faced a number of biases and myths that made adjustment that much more difficult. "I think a lot of people don't understand how difficult it is to gradually, or suddenly, move away from something that was such an integral part of one's personal and professional life." Soon after moving in to this "active adult community," Vernon was at a dinner party and a neighbor said to her, "So, whatever you did in your past life doesn't really matter here; we are all the same." Everyone else sitting around the table nodded in agreement.

"I immediately spoke up," Vernon recalled, "and said that I totally disagreed with this statement. My personal development was intricately related to my professional identity, and that the skills I learned in my careers would continue to play out in my life." Nobody really responded to her after that, but she has found since then there are indeed some prevalent myths and misconceptions that severely limit the ways older people can define their identities. As if to prove her point, Vernon eventually took over responsibilities to organize a charity auction for the community and her leadership skills, honed during many decades as a program chair and leader in the counseling profession, made the event the most successful in a long time. Nevertheless, Vernon feels a lot of pressure from others that she should be "embracing" retirement, playing golf and bridge, maybe doing a little volunteer work.

"They don't understand why I have difficulty letting go of a career I loved, and still do, and that's why I want to continue to do professional things. I realize that a lot of people live for retirement and don't want anything else to do that connects them with that past. On the other hand, I want to make a difference in people's lives—and the best way for me to do that is to do what I know best, which is counseling."

It is particularly frustrating to Vernon the ways that older people continue to be marginalized, based on myths and misconceptions that are not only perpetuated by the culture at large, but even among her contemporaries. "I will never forget attending my first national conference after I retired and a professional associate came up to me and said, 'What are *you* doing here? I thought you had retired.' " She was stunned by that comment, as if she had been told that she no longer belonged at the conference. It felt to her like she had been put out to pasture and told she was no longer valued.

Like so many of her age-mates, Vernon has struggled with trying to find some role and meaning in her so-called retirement. She continues to do workshops and pro bono work with low-income clients. "In all honesty, this has been one of the most difficult transitions of my life. People would say to me that I should do what I love most, but I was already doing that." Because of her passion for counseling, she never had many other hobbies or interests. She worked so much because she truly loved what she was doing.

"When I first retired," Vernon explained, "I tried joining some clubs and other activities. But I was not only bored, but somewhat depressed." She realized that perhaps she had made a mistake quitting her job, but she had felt pressure to do so because her husband was older and ready to do so. Yet she doesn't believe in regrets, so she tried to move forward and make the best of her new situation. This challenge continues to be difficult for her, but she is using all her previous knowledge, wisdom, and skills to make the best of this life stage and reinvent herself once again.

JON: WHEN IS GOING SLOW TOO SLOW?

I have had a very difficult time slowing down and adjusting the pace of my life to a healthy level. I have found that I need to take time off and spend a day or two doing nothing. Until recently, I had never looked at the weekend as a time of rest and recovery, but rather saw it as a time to try to do even more because these were the days that I could do what I really wanted to do. Now I have no real choice. If I cannot rest on the weekend, I really cannot function during the week. I find myself too tired and unable to focus on the issues at hand. When I lament to my age-mates, they all say that is because we are old. I wonder if this is really true? I can't really tell because I got sick at the same time I seemed to have gotten old. Aging seems to be so individual. I have a friend 10 years older than me who says he has never felt better, as he wins yet another triathlon gold medal for his age group. I have another friend a few years younger than me who will only walk around the block so he doesn't get too far from his house in case he has any problems. These two cases remind me that I fit somewhere in the middle.

BIASES AND MISCONCEPTIONS THAT MAY PERMEATE OUR PROFESSION

One of the problems with assessing and exploring older clients' state of well-being is that the language and concepts used better reflect the priorities and developmental tasks of midlife rather than this distinctly different era that can't be understood meaningfully in terms of aspiration and attainment (Hazan, 2011). Elderly people are thus held to standards of productivity and engagement that don't apply to them, and have little relevance to a reshaped identity that has long abandoned the values and priorities of the dominant younger culture. In addition, even the field of gerontology uses terms to describe older people's behavior such as *rolelessness, disintegration, role exit, invisibility,* and *deculturation,* all of which imply a sense of aimlessness and disengagement from what is considered meaningful daily life (Hazan, 1994).

It turns out that happiness and subjective well-being can be defined very differently for older clients. Philosophers have been debating for millennia what exactly constitutes so-called happiness, whether it represents the hedonistic pursuit of pleasure and attainment of goals, or whether instead it means attaining a life that feels meaningful. Obviously, youth and corporate cultures would emphasize the former, and that is one reason why they are held at such a high standard.

Much of the research on subjective well-being flies in the face of many unchallenged assumptions—in particular, that such variables as income level (beyond a minimal level), education, marital status, and even health are the best indicators of life satisfaction. Instead, it seems that one's self-perceptions, attitudes, and personality characteristics matter a whole lot more, which is very good news for those of us who are in the business of helping people to upgrade and enhance those traits and skills (Bormans, 2010; Diener, 2009; Haybron, 2008; Lyubomirsky, 2013; Post, 2005; Seligman, 2011). And even more surprising, it turns out that, with advancing age, one's subjective experience of happiness remains stable and does not decrease despite health-related challenges, losses of loved ones and sensory faculties, and associated mobility issues (Shmotkin, 2011).

If the positive psychology movement has taught us anything during the past few decades it is that therapists should be more focused on virtues, individual resources, and signature strengths of clients, instead of dealing only with innumerable complaints and problems. Of course, clients in general, and older clients in particular, seem to enjoy unloading all their difficulties and frustrations during sessions, and it is easy to feel sorry for them. Through the vital lens of younger therapists, in particular, older clients may appear deserving of our pity, considering their infirmities and decrepitude.

Subjective well-being is not just one structural reality; rather, it is composed of one's private self-awareness, publically declared condition, and the dominant narrative or story that has been internalized. Some clients tell us they are perfectly miserable, they have nothing left to live for, and they have been abandoned and put out to pasture, but that declarative subjective well-being does not necessarily reflect what is experienced on a daily basis (Shmotkin, 2005). What could be more fun that regaling some know-it-all "youngster" with stories about how tough it is to get out of bed in the morning or to get one's son or daughter to return calls?

As therapists age, it is likely that our levels of compassion and understanding will also grow. For example, the importance of reminiscing and living in the past, the topic of our next chapter, will be better understood and appreciated. This seems to be a time of immense change in terms of our understanding and appreciating these final life stages. Now that large numbers of Baby Boomers have hit their 70s, much more interest is being shown for what is actual and possible.

CHAPTER 8
Living in the Past

Those who love deeply never grow old; they may die of old age, but they die young.
Ben Franklin

One of the myths and misconceptions of aging is that it is often perceived that, because older people appear to be so idle, depressed, lonely, and unproductive, they spend most of their time living in the past. They talk way too much about the "good ole days" and continually criticize young people for their recklessness and lack of respect. Although this might actually be the case for a minority of elderly who do indeed have little going for them in the present, as we've seen, the vast majority of those in later life lead full and productive lives.

There has never been a time in human history when cultural and technological advancements occur so quickly, making our tools and devices virtually obsolete within a few years. It is also true that, with age, it does become more challenging to adapt to rapid changes when it seems that things were working just fine the way they were. Whether we are speaking about new cellular devices, software updates, or therapeutic approaches on the scene, there may come a time when there is a cry from the, older generation, "Enough is enough!"

Indeed, many of us who have been practicing for several decades become cynical, and perhaps even resistant, to supposed innovative models that already seem familiar, even if couched in new language. When one feels perfectly comfortable operating in a time-tested and refined approach that appears to work quite well, there is less than enthusiastic glee over the prospect of learning a whole new system that requires considerable time and effort to master.

THE GOOD OL' DAYS

We remember during the heyday of relatively long-term therapy when it was simply expected that clients would spend many months, if not years, in treatment to do legitimate, solid work. It probably helped us to think that way, considering we were in private practice, rewarded for this belief.

This was a time when insurance companies routinely covered 90% of whatever was charged, with sessions scheduled as often as desirable and no lifetime limit. You'd have to have been crazy not to be in therapy. And it is no wonder that older therapists long for those bygone days when we had so much more discretion and power to structure therapy in ways we thought were most advantageous for our clients (and for ourselves).

We know we aren't the only ones over 50 who feel this way, even as the field has moved dramatically into a direction of offering brief interventions following manualized, empirically supported treatments. It is ironic that Nicholas Cummings, now in his 90s and still professionally active, was one of the architects of managed care as chief psychologist for Kaiser Permanente, one of the largest mental health organizations on the planet. Before he served as president of the American Psychological Association, he worked tirelessly for a half century to advocate on behalf of therapists to work in primary healthcare settings alongside physicians and other medical professionals.

Cummings resents that he is viewed as an "elder psychotherapist, without the realization we are the generation that literally established the profession from scratch. As the history of psychology is no longer taught in grad school, they are unaware of the difficulties, battles and misunderstandings involved in developing a profession they think has always been there." By "they," Cummings is referring mostly to younger professionals who seem oblivious to the foundation that was established by their seniors.

In a similar vein, Cummings feels wistful about the way things used to be versus the current, limited status of the field. "I find today's practice lacking the vitality that was fervent in the early days," he admits. "This is when we were establishing the practice against all odds, such as psychiatric opposition, absence of licensure, and third-party payment, as well as little societal recognition. In other words, the exciting pioneer spirit no longer exists."

Of course Cummings is correct that the pioneer days are over, just as they end whenever a profession or movement matures into the next stages of development. He recalls during the 1970s when the practice of therapy was limited to doctoral-level professionals, whereas now there are so many more masters-level therapists. Of course it was also during the 1970s when our own masters degrees consisted of 30 credit hours when now it is more than double the amount and depth of training and preparation.

There have been a number of other changes that Cummings and his contemporaries have witnessed throughout the years, many of them viewed as a big step backward. "Even though psychodynamics have purged itself from Freudian mumbo-jumbo, psychotherapy is essentially limited to [cognitive–behavioral therapy]. Although cognitive–behavioral strategies are important and useful, they are only a part of what psychotherapy should be." Cummings is both disappointed and annoyed that, although cognitive approaches are helpful in correcting faulty thinking, they virtually ignore causation and instead remain focused on empirically validating specific techniques.

Cummings insists he does not look back, but looks forward. "I remain young and on the cutting edge. I have my health and I am still vigorous. I am proud that I have *finally* tumbled onto the realization that the mainstream will always be behind and that I can create outside the establishment. More than ever I am aware of what Steve Jobs meant when he said that people don't know what they want until we show them."

Robert Wubbolding, a prominent theorist and promoter of reality therapy, is insistent that it's far more useful to leave the past behind and move on. He has learned from experience that it isn't all that helpful to talk about the "good ole days," much less remain stuck in them. He finds nostalgia mostly boring, if not off-putting, especially to those who are younger. Most of us remember, during our younger days, being bored to distraction by old people who kept telling us that nothing today comes close to how things used to be during simpler times—those that have been overidealized and romanticized.

Wubbolding loves to tell stories, especially those based on his varied experiences. Most people are surprised to learn that during an earlier incarnation he was Catholic priest before he became a secular therapist. He also thrives on new innovations in the field and stays current on the latest advances in neuroscience. He has also long been interested in reading and studying widely way outside the field of therapy, and this has helped to keep him fresh and energized. "I see many possible ways for these interests to interface with counseling and therapy. For instance, a book that has impacted me over the years, and one that I read every few years, is *The Divine Milieu* by Teilhard de Chardin, a philosopher, anthropologist, and theologian. He believed that all our actions contribute to the evolution of humankind and retain an eternal existence. This is an encouraging concept for therapists who meet people on a very deep level and help them to make better choices, thereby adding to the *pleroma*, or fullness, toward which we are all evolving."

Wubbolding has also avoided living in the past—except for occasional lapses—by connecting more deeply in his current relationships with his wife, family members, colleagues, friends, students, clients, and workshop participants. "This impact has taught me about personal responsibility, the responsibility for relating to people in a sensitive and yet honest manner, and that the words we use make a difference in the lives of people. I came to realize the significance of these ideas early in my career as a professional person. As a Catholic priest, I realized that words could help or hurt. When used by a person respected in the community—clergy, therapist, politician, parent, employer, medical professional, and, in fact, anyone—they *can* touch a person deeply, even to the point where the listeners change their life."

SIGMUND FREUD'S LAST DAYS

When we think about historical figures from the past who created and shaped what psychotherapy has become, Freud's name has got to jump to the top of the list. Although he borrowed ideas from a number of other philosophers, physicians, collaborators, students, and novelists, more than anyone else he can be credited with "inventing" the earliest version of the "helping cure."

It would appear that most of Freud's groundbreaking work occurred before he turned 50, yet he kept reinventing himself over and over again throughout his lifetime, delving into anthropology, archaeology, mythology, sociology, as well as his beloved neurology. In a remarkable piece of research about Freud's last year, Edmundson (2007) followed an almost day-by-day progression of the great man's failing health and struggle to come to terms with his aging identity and eventual death. Freud was a scandalous dreamer, a revolutionary thinker, and a challenger of authority and the status quo never more than during his final years. Here's a guy who proposed that infants have erotic desires, that boys want to have sex with their mothers and kill their fathers, that even jokes and slips of the tongue reveal hidden desires. He told the world that we are all hedonists driven to the pursuit of pleasure and submission to authority, motivated by forces beyond our awareness.

As an older man in his 80s, Freud was in constant pain from cancer that had invaded his mouth and was eating away at his jaw. He was exhausted, depressed, and despairing at all the losses he experienced. His sisters perished in Nazi concentration camps. He eventually lost his vision and ability to speak. He lost his country to Hitler and had to flee his homeland during a time he could barely walk. Yet it was his work that kept him going.

Freud didn't exactly complete his best work during these later years, but he remained very active professionally. And he did so with the self-centered indulgence of an old man. He had long ago required his patients to lie on a couch, not to facilitate better free association, but because he didn't like being stared at all day. He smoked his foul-smelling cigars, fogging up the room, and allowing his dog, Yofi, to run wild during sessions. One of his patients remarked, "I felt the professor was more interested in Yofi than he was in my story" (Dolittle, 1956, p. 162).

During his last year in Vienna, Freud closed his practice and stopped seeing patients because he felt too distracted. Between the Nazi invasion as an external factor, and his own declining health and chronic pain, he could no longer focus on sessions with appropriate attention. Following his own prescription, he observed that "when the conscious mind is troubled, one cannot be interested in the unconscious mind" (Molnar, 1992, p. 233). He was troubled indeed.

Letting go of his profession as a therapist was another tremendous loss, only adding to his depression and deterioration, "cutting him off from what was probably his major source of inspiration as a writer and thinker" (Edmundson, 2007, pp. 105–106). Afterward he struggled with boredom and continuing meaningful work, often taking long naps on his famous couch.

Even the most formidable personalities and esteemed therapists struggle with the adjustments required to accept the inevitable declining health and frustrations of aging. After losses to his hearing, vision, speech, and mobility, Freud surrendered to despair at times, wishing for an end. "I cannot reconcile myself to the wretchedness and helplessness of being old, and look forward to the transition into nonbeing with a kind of longing" (Gay, 1971, p. 162).

During the last weeks of Freud's life, he was literally decomposing. There was a huge crater open on the side of his face from which a horrible odor emanated. Gangrene had set in and flies swarmed around him on a death watch. Even his beloved dog sat cowering in the corner, appalled by the awful smell. In one of his last letters he described himself as a "small island of pain floating on an ocean of indifference." He then chose the moment of his death, having struck a deal with his physician to administer a lethal dose of morphine. He died on his own terms just as he lived.

Freud had plenty of time to come to terms with his own death after living with a cancer diagnosis for more than 15 years. It was important to him that he leave this world with dignity. Yet he rallied after relocating to England for his last year. He resumed seeing patients again. He worked furiously to complete his last major project, perhaps one of his most provocative of all—*Moses and Monotheism*. He proposed the rather controversial idea that the prophet who led the Jews out of slavery was actually an Egyptian nobleman. Furthermore, that it was regret over the murder of their leader that led Jews thereafter to seek religion to appease their guilt.

The public outcry and critical response invigorated rather than discouraged Freud. Edmundson (2007) believes that the reactions made Freud feel young again, up to his old mischief of turning people's beliefs upside down. He loved that he was stirring up as much trouble as he had in his youth, even when his friends and colleagues petitioned him to not publish the book. "Quite a worthy exit," Freud remarked.

With a temporary burst of renewed energy, Freud enjoyed seeing patients again. He received an assortment of prominent visitors who made a pilgrimage to pay homage to him—Salvador Dali, Virginia Woolf, H. G. Wells, and an assortment of dignitaries, scientists, political figures, and even the Nazi official who held him captive in Austria. It was a time in life, his final stage, when he very much focused on the past and his legacy. And yes, he eventually became quite crotchety, demanding, and difficult to deal with—understandably so given his constant suffering and discomfort.

BRINGING THE PAST INTO THE PRESENT

Older clients aren't the only ones who live in the past. We could make a case that many of the issues that are brought to us involve people who can't let go of things that continue to haunt them. They obsess about past slights and injustices. They remain stuck in habitual behavior that plagues them. They continue to subscribe to beliefs and attitudes that, although singularly counterproductive, remain guiding forces in their life.

Memories and reminiscences are what make connections between what we once were and what we are now. As such, they serve important functions to help create meaning from our life and provide a context for daily experiences. Contrary to the common belief, most older people do not generally spend more time daydreaming about the past than younger people, although it may seem that way because they have so much more territory to cover.

Reminiscences among the elderly are also not necessarily about nostalgia or escaping the present into the past, but rather they can often represent a constructive process of life review, as well as a resolution of unfinished business. In some cases, such explorations of the past may even act as an immunity to depression and discouragement (Moody & Sasser, 2015).

Angus was in his early 80s when he showed up for his first session. He was having some recent challenges with his memory and what seemed like depression, which was especially upsetting for his daughter, who insisted he seek help for his problems. "My father has always been a very private person," she explained on the phone while setting up his first appointment. "I must admit that I don't really know him very well."

It was apparent during the first session that Angus was indeed not the most expressive or articulate person. He wasn't really sure why he was there, nor could he think about anything that he really wanted—or needed—to talk about. He responded to each question with a shrug or a single-word answer.

His therapist decided to provide more structure for the conversation that didn't seem to be going anywhere. He launched into a careful review of life history, hoping to discover something useful, and he immediately noticed that Angus perked up when he started talking about his early life. What unfolded was a beautiful story of a hard-working man who, with the help of a close-knit family, had overcome many obstacles to reach a level of relative success and satisfaction.

Angus talked with pride about his hard-working immigrant father who wanted his children to be successful. His father had a job at the local dairy and eventually became a part owner and manager. There were eight children in the family, including Angus, so there was a certain amount of drama in the house at all times. Angus disclosed that he was required to drop out of school at age 13 to go to work, and he told the story of how he first met his wife of 55 years. He described his friends, work, children, grandchildren, and hobbies, and he was deeply touched by all that he had been able to do in his life.

As Angus recalled vacations and camping trips with his family, he began to talk with even more passion. He described fishing trips, baseball games, catching frogs and butterflies, and swimming. He described how they were eventually able to purchase some land on a lake and build a cabin that had now grown to be a house and the family gathering place each summer. It was as if his life mattered a little more with each session and each story he shared.

When Angus was asked why he was viewed as such a private and withholding person by his daughter, given how loquacious he was talking about his life experiences, he just kind of shrugged. "I didn't think she was all that interested in my story."

BRINGING HISTORY ALIVE

In the context of later life, the functions of storytelling are part of the evolutionary role to pass on lessons to younger generations. Traditionally, this took the form of teaching younger members of the tribe about fertile hunting grounds, triumphs and failures, and moral values; more recently in human history, it often represents meaning making. For instance, so often supervision by senior therapists takes the form of recollection about seminal events in the history of our profession or interactions with some of the significant figures.

The Evolution of Psychotherapy conferences held every five years, as well as other international events, gather the field's greatest minds, or at least those that are most self-promoting, to pass along their wisdom and experience to the next generation of therapists. We have been privileged to interview more than 100 prominent theorists during the past decade, and Jon has produced hundreds of videos profiling their work in action. Through these conference presentations and dialogues, interviews, videos, and case examples presented in several previous volumes, we have tried to act as a conduit between the history of our past and the cutting edge of contemporary therapeutic work.

The old adage that those who are not familiar with mistakes of the past are doomed to repeat them is certainly true with respect to supposed innovations in our field. Anyone who has been in practice long enough can easily become cynical about supposedly new innovations in the field that are simply repackaged ideas with new names that seem more designed to earn the author notoriety than actually to increase our knowledge.

Despite significant advancements in empirically validated treatments and evidence-based practice, there are certain standard operating principles that have been true in the past and are still true today. One of these dimensions that holds special meaning when working with older clients is the critical importance of remaining fully present during the interaction, even when conversation is very much about the past. This is the case even though some elderly clients may live in a state of "dreamland," or an alternative reality as a function of memory problems or dementia; it is just as important, if not more so, to remain as fully present as possible during sessions. It is this complete engagement that can help them to remain focused and attuned: "presence provides a bridge from the dreamland state back to consensus reality" (Suri, 2010, p. 177).

Some of the most prominent existential writers in the field, such as Yalom (1980) and Bugental (1985), felt that nothing was more important than being fully present with clients, never more so than in the latter stages of their own lives. We recall interviewing Bugental at age 87, shortly before he died (Kottler & Carlson, 2003)—a time when he was struggling with some cognitive and memory issues. He had "lost" a lot of his past and found it difficult to recall much about some aspects of his work, but he still remained passionately committed to the power of relationships. In his soft, gentle voice he talked about a case in which a black man approached him for treatment to make him white. He couldn't remember much about what he said or did with the man, but he started to become emotional as he talked about the case.

"Yes, he was a very dear man," Bugental said. "I grew very attached to him. I was so sorry that I was not able to help him more. That was. . . I feel a little choked up right now just remembering him. It was such a hard thing for him to finally accept himself that he was black and would always be black" (Kottler & Carlson, 2003, p. 278). It is this strong connection to those he helped that remained with him until his last breath.

We found Bugental's story especially moving and profound, not so much because of the case itself, but rather because it was so apparent how deeply he cared about his clients. During a time when there is so much emphasis on exactly which diagnosis is chosen, which corresponding interventions are selected, which assessment tools are chosen, and which outcome measures are used, it feels like such an important reminder from the past to concentrate on *being with* our clients with body, mind, heart, and soul.

CHAPTER 9

Common Issues and Challenges of the Elderly

Not much is done for old people in our culture. . . . Many persons seem to be changed when they are older, and this is mainly due to the fact that they feel futile and useless. Then they try to improve their worth and value again in the same way as adolescents do. They interfere and want to show in many ways that they are not old and will not be overlooked, or else they become disappointed and depressed.

Alfred Adler

It is certainly obvious that working with elderly clients presents some special challenges unlike any others we might face in therapy. There are often complicated medical conditions, including both an extensive history and perhaps a number of medications involved; each brings its own side effects. There are usually some fairly ingrained family patterns, many of which may act to compromise any change efforts. And then there are the possibly diminished capacities of the very old to respond to treatment effectively. In the words of one client who challenged his therapist: "I'm 95, depressed, unable to walk, tired, in pain, and have nothing to look forward to. I'm going to die soon anyway. What can you possibly do for me?" (Agronin, 2010, p. 101).

In facing the almost overwhelming challenges of such a case, the therapist can't help but shrug in agreement, if not despair. There is no quick cure for such a case, no simple solution that restores the client to previous levels of functioning. And yet, we can expect more older clients than ever to seek help for their most frequent complaints, which may include difficulties coping with their current living situation, adjustment and accommodation to losses, lack of social support, conflicts with family members, physical illnesses, disabilities, and chronic pain. And of course there is also coming to terms with impending death.

THE FUTURE OF THERAPY

More than ever before, people are seeking therapeutic experiences as they age. In part, this is the result of the Baby Boomer cohort that has always been committed to seeking forms of enlightenment, whether transcendental meditation and encounter groups of the 1960s or new incarnations that have come to pass since then. Yet people of all backgrounds and eras, living longer than ever before, are searching for opportunities to reflect on the meaning of their life. One 83-year-old man had never considered therapy previously, but after his wife died and his business partnership ended, he realized he needed something more than just hanging out with his grandchildren. "I don't know how long I'm going to live," he said, "but I want to make it easier. Everybody needs help, and everybody makes mistakes. I needed to reach outside my own capabilities" (Ellin, 2013).

Therapists who were interviewed in this article by Ellin about their experiences working with elderly clients revealed they are seeing increasing interest among older people to seek help. In some cases, they have unfinished business they wish to work through or want assistance with some troublesome area of their lives. Also, many people in their 80s and older are neither depressed nor miserable, but reach out to therapists for support, companionship, social interaction, or stimulating conversation. They have jettisoned the belief that they are too old to change.

This stands in stark contrast to the number of younger therapists who may continue to hold ageist beliefs that pathologize the normal development of older adults although they actually are *less* likely to manifest mental disorders (Narrow, Rae, Robins, & Regier, 2002). Tomko and Munley (2013) highlighted some of the most common negative attitudes, which result primarily from a lack of training and exposure to this population. We've mentioned the neglect in this area previously—that although it is required to have courses and supervised experience in child therapy, it is somewhat more rare to have similar preparation with older adults. Similarly, although there is mandated curricular offerings in multicultural sensitivity and diverse populations, this is most often focused on gender, ethnicity, and religious diversity rather than age cohorts as distinctive cultures with their own norms, rituals, language, and needs. It is perhaps not surprising that the closer in age therapists are to their older clients, the less likely they are to hold such biases.

SOME OF OUR MOST CHALLENGING CLIENTS

There is no doubt that some of the most complex and difficult cases we will ever handle may very well involve older clients. At every age and stage of life, there are particular kinds of issues, complaints, and client characteristics that test our patience and push us to the limits of what we can do. With respect to elderly clients, there are certainly some especially frustrating individuals, including those who ramble a lot and repeat themselves constantly. We will encounter those with rigid beliefs and attitudes, believing they are too old to change, giving in to discouragement and despair that feels contagious. There are clients who present chronic and intractable pain and suffering, and complain about their discomfort—a lot. There are those who are so overmedicated that addressing their various complaints and maladies doesn't appear to have the slightest chance of penetrating their stupor. And there are those with serious cognitive impairment or dementia who may not be good candidates for therapy in the first place because of their inability to follow threads of conversation.

Glicken (2009) has categorized many of the most common challenges of aging adults. These include those that involve love and intimacy issues, ageism and discrimination in the workplace, retirement stress, social isolation and loneliness, elder abuse and neglect, depression and suicidal ideation, anxiety related to issues of uncertainty and certainty (death), terminal illnesses and chronic pain, spiritual and religious issues, dementia and cognitive deterioration, disabilities and adaptation to assisted living, and bereavement, grief, and loss. We mention several of these that are most difficult to handle.

Transference Issues

Many therapists are uncomfortable with the difficult and chronic problems of their aging clients. What do we do for chronic pain that has no cure? How do we really resolve difficulties that involve devastating disabilities, degenerative illnesses, major cognitive deterioration, and losses that may involve almost everything that was once familiar? Many of us got into this field in the first place because we so desperately need to fix problems. Needless to say, it is quite challenging for us to accept, sometimes, the realistic limits of what we can do, and that it often seems like it is not nearly enough. It may trigger our own sense of helplessness, not to mention our own terrors associated with growing older.

As we know, transference-type reactions often occur in both directions between therapists and clients. Our older clients imagine us in particular ways, associate us with others they have known, or, in some cases, may write us off because of our perceived youth and inexperience. Likewise, many of our older clients remind us of figures from the past, both benevolent and adversarial. In both cases, these projections create additional challenges that can be compounded if they are not fully recognized and understood.

Without awareness of the issues, or supervision to monitor reactions, much distortion and possible harm can occur during the therapeutic process. Common distortions involve the therapist being identified as a child, grandchild, parent, spouse at an early age, an erotic object, or as a social authority figure (Knight,

JEFFREY: TRIGGERING MY OWN TERROR

I will volunteer to be among the first to admit that I became a therapist because of my early experiences with feeling so helpless and out of control. I yearned for ways that I might regain some kind stability, some sense of hope that I didn't have to feel like a victim of circumstances outside of my control. And I did indeed find the answer to my quest when I trained to become a therapist, learning all kinds of ways to resolve difficulties, fix problems, and, yes, cure chronic issues that had once seemed intractable. The most "fun" I ever have as a therapist is when I find ways that a client and I can answer perplexing questions or, better yet, actually make things so much better. And I love it when we can do that relatively quickly. So it has been my lifelong struggle to sit with people when I realize there are no easy answers and really no cures for what they present. My frustration and impatience kick in, triggering once again my own feelings of helplessness and forcing me to realize that I really don't have as much control as I pretend I do. It is sometimes terrifying.

2004). Therapists must be cautious about interacting with their older clients in a manner that could lead to their own unresolved issues and situations.

Therapists might also have memories of, or associations with, elders who were strong or weak, kind or irritable, supportive or demanding, loving or cold, involved or uninvolved. We may have feelings of pity, deference, love, guilt, worship, anger, or sadness associated with elders (Kampfe, 2014). These thoughts and feelings might influence our thoughts and feelings about our current clients. It is important to assess honestly any issues they may have with elders or any societal ageist perspectives to ensure we do not influence our therapy with older clients (Kampfe, 2014). And others strongly recommend that we should not work with older clients until these unresolved thoughts and feelings are resolved.

Body Changes

How do you feel good about your appearance when your most prominent features—hair color, skin texture, posture, and body shape—are all in need of repair or rejuvenation? Hair dye, toupees and wigs, dental or hair implants, cosmetic creams, girdles, Botox injections, wardrobe, even surgery, can try to disguise or hide natural changes, but the reality remains that only youth is really considered attractive.

Despite all the efforts designed to make the body appear younger, there are also fears that are very much grounded in reality. Older people may often restrict activities or limit movement because of fears of falling—a circumstance that younger people don't often fully appreciate. In fact, the consequence of taking a fall after age 65 can be catastrophic for the individual, often resulting in a broken hip from more fragile bones. More than one-third of seniors do take a tumble each year, making for a high probability of injury. The consequence of a broken hip, despite surgical repairs, means that more than half these individuals will end up with limited mobility and never walk as well again. Even more frightening is that 40% will land in a nursing home as a result, and 37% of them will end up dead within a year (Gillick, 2006).

The aging process of the older adult appears to be the exact opposite of adolescents and children. All the things that were happening during the early stages of life are operating quite differently. As young children we go through a process that involves standing up, walking with support, and then being able to walk alone. During the end of life that scenario is reversed. Learning to accept this decline is important, as well as making necessary adjustments that capitalize on mobility strengths. That's why therapists who work with this population often prescribe activities such as yoga, stretching, and other regular movement exercises.

Mental Decline

One would never guess that Leita, a very active, vibrant woman in her 70s, engaged in all kinds of community service and art projects, takes care of her sick husband and keeps her losses mostly to herself. When asked about the greatest challenge she has noticed, she immediately blurted out, "Memory loss! Yikes!"

Leita had always considered her extraordinary memory to be her greatest gift. "But now during conversations, the names and words are not just there. I have always played memory games with myself, word associations, visualizations, and now I freeze and feel frustrated." She also lost the sight in one of her eyes, leading her to feel even more handicapped. And that's not the end of what she has noticed. "I can't swim as far. I don't ice skate anymore for fear of falling and hurting myself and breaking something. I wasn't exactly fearless before, but now I am much more cautious."

As mentioned, you would never guess that Leita feels such fear, apprehension, or mourns any losses, because she appears so active and engaged in everything she does. Like most successful older adults she has learned to compensate and adapt to the changes she has experienced with her memory difficulties or slower cognitive processing.

As we have discussed, memory loss and some reduction in cognitive functioning are inevitable with aging. This can range from a minor reduction in mental alertness to major Alzheimer symptoms in which a person can't even function very well without close supervision.

It is often challenging to figure out whether memory difficulties are the result of normal cognitive decline associated with aging, symptoms of dementia, or evidence of an underlying mood disorder. There are assessment procedures often used to make this differential diagnosis, many of which look at behavioral deficits, including the following:

- Forgets appointments, commitments, or significant dates (holidays, birthdays)
- Repeats the same questions or statements repeatedly
- Demonstrates difficulty remembering recent events
- Forgets names of friends and family members
- Loses interest in lifelong activities, hobbies, and social activities
- Displays unpredictable agitation, irritability, or mood fluctuations
- Becomes lost while driving or walking
- Can no longer handle daily tasks related to finances, transportation, bathing, or eating

More and more medical facilities are creating memory clinics, where comprehensive assessments are conducted. Memory and other signs of mental decline can often be attributed to prescription side effects, withdrawal from social life, lack of physical exercise, lack of meaning, and other causes similar to those associated with depression. Memory clinics often provide practices that contribute to a healthy brain, including physical exercise, regular mental and intellectual stimulation, social interaction, a healthy diet, plenty of restful sleep, stress management strategies, and low alcohol consumption

Personality Shifts

There are some interesting ways that people's basic nature can evolve with aging, with some people becoming more placid and introverted, and others more assertive and outgoing. Political beliefs and values can become more conservative, just as religious observance can become more significant.

The personal experience of aging is obviously harder for some people than others. Some people have great difficulty growing old, not because of their living context is objectively more difficult or harsh, but because they make assumptions about themselves and their world that highlight the burdens of old age (Hill, 2005). Counselors can be helpful in reducing the impact of rigidity, negativity, worry, self-absorption, and regret (Hill, 2005). Although there are many other personality traits that can be assessed, these are some of the primary ones that can make aging even more difficult.

According to Knight's (2004) review of the available research, the transition to old age for men is usually relatively stable whereas for women it is sometimes a time that signifies considerable reorganization of the personality. Both men and women typically become more introverted, philosophical, and reflective, and even when personality remains stable and consistent, older people tend to believe they have changed a lot. This, of course, makes them particularly good candidates for therapy.

Although almost by definition, personality traits—for the most part—supposedly don't change very much there are some counseling strategies that can modify some of the traits. Older adults seem to want to maintain positive emotions—a task that is accomplished more easily now than other times in life because of greater ability to regulate feelings. Again, this makes them perfect psychotherapy clients.

Isolation and Social Engagement

We have said earlier that older people are not necessarily more lonely than younger people; in some ways, with lowered expectations for relationships, they may even feel more satisfied. Social networks shrink quite naturally as people become more selective as they age, more inclined to spend time in quality relationships rather than trying to maintain a large quantity of friendships. Intimacy because more precious. You can observe this readily in social media in which young people often keep score to collect as many contacts and "friends" as possible whereas older participants are content with fewer, more limited connections.

It is also the case that friends die and lose contact over time, increasing the risk of social isolation, which is a predictor of poor health. There is some evidence, in fact, that immune systems may become compromised among those who lose social contact with others (Carstensen, 2011). The encouraging news, however, is that older people need fewer relationships to feel satisfied. Although, they tend to spend more time alone, they become much more comfortable with solitude and feel less need to be around others just for the sake of companionship.

In one interesting and surprising study the researchers counted the frequency of relational words used in people's autobiographies, such as *friend, brother,* and *sister*; and plural pronouns such as *we* and *us*. Incredibly, they found that those with a greater number of relational references actually lived five years longer than those with fewer such references. This appeared to demonstrate the importance of social engagement in maintaining health and life satisfaction, as well as increasing longevity.

It would appear that three is the magic number in terms of the ideal number of ongoing intimate relationships for older people. This strikes a balance between codependency on one family member or friend, and too many relationships to maintain a high level of personal contact. Carstensen (2011) believes this is the result of "socioemotional selectivity" in that older people feel less motivated to create new relationships and are more inclined to maintain the few connections that are already most satisfying and supportive. She also notes how the very structure of families is evolving. It used to be quite rare that grandparents, much less great-grandparents, existed; in the future, it will be quite common to have four-generation or even five-generation families. And then with the relatively common occurrence of divorce and remarriage, gay marriage, multiple sets of parents and grandparents, blended families, multiple-hyphenated names and identities, some interesting challenges will be presented for therapists in helping their clients navigate through these complexities.

There are five basic questions that need to be addressed when feeling lonely, regardless of one's age. It is more complex than just finding three people to call friends. Counselors can help their older clients to assess their responses and to see where they most need to focus.

1. *Figure out who you are.* Help clients to identify those characteristics that represent their core values, the attributes that define them. Encourage them to translate these ideals into action every day. If they wish to be known as a kind person, then help them to commit to practicing kindness on a daily basis. Of course, such behavior also invites others to draw closer.
2. *Invest in connections to other people.* Texting, e-mailing, and social media don't have quite the same impact as face-to-face intimacy that builds ongoing support.
3. *Get involved in the community—globally or locally.* Investing time, money, and energy in people outside one's social circle not only helps create a sense of meaning and achievement, but also facilitates closer connections to others.
4. *Channel talents into meaningful work.* Volunteer work, mentioned earlier, can be just as satisfying as paid employment—assuming that economic realities don't intrude.
5. *Take time to figure out what is most important.* Make sure everyday habits are representative of your one's purpose. As time becomes more limited, more precious, it is important to have conversations about how to invest one's energy in those activities that are more satisfying and useful.

Lifestyle Issues

A big part of our job assisting older adults has less to do with what we talk about in sessions and a lot more that is related to what we can help them to do differently in their daily lives. Although we could say the same thing about anyone in therapy, it is even more important with this population. A century or two ago the

JEFFREY: WHAT IT MEANS TO BE "PRODUCTIVE" AS WE AGE

I had so much work left to do—papers to read and grade, articles to review, messages to respond to, administrative chores to complete, travel reservations to make, and this dang book to complete. Oh yeah, I also had to get ready for the next morning's packed schedule, and figure out what to wear and what I'd need to bring with me. Oh! And I was two episodes behind on one of my favorite television shows, and the DVR would erase them out of spite if I didn't take care of that unfinished business.

There was a spectacular storm outside, lightening raced across the sky and the thunder was so powerful I could feel its vibrations in my feet. My two-year-old granddaughter is terrified of thunder and so she grabbed onto my legs and wouldn't let go as I headed to my study. Crap. So much to do and so little time.

But I had just written this section about how older people become much more discerning about their priorities, and that led me to consider what was really most important to me in that moment: getting work done or literally holding my granddaughter. I nodded my head because things were really so clear to me.

We went outside on the covered patio and Aliya stretched out on my lap as we watched the lightning sparkle like fireworks. Every time it thundered we'd both scream and yell and clap our hands. We screamed for more. We did a thunder dance. And I can't recall a more meaningful and important half hour that I've ever spent in my life. Screw the work.

major causes of death were pneumonia, smallpox, and influenza; nowadays they are cancer, heart disease, and stroke—all of which are directly related to lifestyle issues such as exercise, diet, smoking, and other daily habits (Carstensen, 2011).

For those older adults who do end up in therapy, Woodhead, Ivan, and Emery (2013) asked 50 clients about their motivations for seeking treatment. The most common reason mentioned, by more than half the participants, was depression. This was especially the case for those who were dealing with significant losses. The second most common reason cited was the motivation to improve their lives as a result of seeing others their age do the same. Family conflicts were also a factor for many of the clients, with one of them mentioning, for example, that among his five children, only one of them was actually speaking to him. Health concerns were also commonly expressed as a reason for entering therapy, such as those instances when the person was fearful about upcoming surgery, struggling with a disease, or worried about death. Finally, about 20% began treatment for reasons similar to anyone else; they wanted to increase self-awareness or understand themselves better.

With regard to this last incentive to begin therapy, although there have been many existing biases and beliefs that insight-oriented, long-term therapy is not appropriate for older adults because, as Freud originally noted, they are too rigid and impervious to change, one longitudinal study of elderly clients in psychodynamic therapy found they profited significantly from exploring many of the same unresolved issues that would be addressed by anyone else (Roseborough, Luptak, McLeod, & Bradshaw, 2013).

When the Cure Is the Problem

People older than 65 are responsible for half of all drug prescriptions (Hall, 2001). One reason for this, which is hardly surprising, is they are more susceptible to chronic health conditions—arthritis, high blood pressure, heart disease, and cancer. But another compelling reason, and one just as important, is the attitude of the medical profession toward elderly patients who present symptoms of depression, loneliness, anxiety, pain, or compromised life satisfaction. More often than not they will leave a doctor's office with a prescription. Add to that the pharmaceutical industry now spends more on marketing drugs than they do on their actual research and product development.

The result is that the majority of elderly people are taking drugs they don't actually need—and can't afford—to comply with medical treatment. Many doctors don't consider, much less explore, the underlying need and desire for older patients simply to talk about what is bothering them. This is no less the case with almost anyone who seeks medical consultation, considering the average amount of time a patient has the chance to talk about a presenting problem is 18 seconds before he or she is interrupted, and only 1 in 50 patients is ever given the chance to finish his or her story before being dismissed (Levine, 2004).

For those older people living in nursing homes, it is sometimes the case that three-quarters of the residents are given sedatives and sleeping pills—regardless of whether they need them. According to the physicians who routinely prescribe them, the stated attitude is often that, at their age, the side effects and addictive properties of the drugs don't matter much (Flick, Garms-Homolova, & Rohnsch, 2012). It isn't surprising, then, that most older adults fill at least a dozen prescriptions each year, and that one-fifth routinely use pain medications (Wilson et al., 2007).

Family Members and Caregivers

What goes around comes around, so to speak. Just as we all begin life in diapers, many of us end up wearing them as life ends. As we mentioned earlier, it is strange to consider that, in Japan, there is more of a demand for adult diapers than those for infants because the population is aging so quickly. Likewise, just as our earliest years required caregivers to meet our basic needs and keep us safe, so, too, do many older people require assistance from family members and hired staff. This presents some particular challenges for therapy in that some older clients cannot be treated in isolation (which is the case with almost anyone), but must be viewed within a larger systemic context that includes others intimately involved in their safety and care.

There are, let us say, some rather interesting relational dynamics in many families in which an older member requires considerable assistance. This can range from somewhat minimal care for food preparation or transportation to almost constant monitoring for those experiencing severe dementia or health issues. It is one of the therapist's jobs to assess the quality of care provided, the interrelated web of relationships, as well as any conflicts present.

As we discuss in the next section, the workload and burden that family members may shoulder, especially in the case of an older spouse, can lead to a host of additional problems. Caregivers are known to have much higher rates of mental illness and emotional problems than the general population of the same age; they are more likely to visit doctors, abuse drugs and alcohol, report acute stress and anxiety, and exhibit sleep and appetite problems; and they are three times more likely to be depressed (Agronin, 2010).

BURDENS OF CAREGIVERS

During a period of life when many people over 50 are just beginning to adjust to their own issues related to aging, they take on additional responsibilities related to caring for their elderly parents or relatives. In the case of many women, in particular, they may now spend more time caring for their parents than their children because they are far more likely than men to provide backup assistance for family members who need help (Aronson & Weiner, 2007). This often creates a number of additional stressors that often respond well to therapeutic intervention.

In addition to caring for aging parents, it is inevitable that one elderly partner or spouse will eventually end up having to take care of the other, just at a time when he or she needs support as well. As one example, a woman kept a diary of some of her thoughts and feelings related to taking care of her husband, who had suffered a series of strokes. "It's so hard to contend with something like this, to keep loving someone who calls you names and treats you like an enemy. . . . I also remember how thoughtful he used to be. . . . Now, he's so wrapped up in his own mixed-up world and in his own thoughts, he hardly pays any attention to what's going on around him, or what he's doing" (Shiplett, 1996).

In another case, Karyn, at age 76, struggles with her own medical issues that disrupt her sleep and lead to chronic pain. Because of financial issues, she can't afford to hire extra help for her husband, who is in his 80s and is confined to a wheelchair as a result of a stroke. Because of the nature of his brain damage, his cognitive functioning is severely impaired, and he is extremely emotionally volatile and unpredictable.

Although there are many things that Karyn can't control related to their limited income and resources, in addition to chronic physical limitations, she desperately needs emotional support and reassurance, which has been hard to come by from her own family. A therapist has been absolutely crucial to provide that help, giving her an opportunity to talk about her frustrations and sense of helplessness. A number of studies have validated this experience as quite common, because caregivers consistently report they have rarely shared their stories with others (Sorrell, 2014).

GIFTS AND BURDENS

There is estimated to be more than 65 *million* family caregivers in the United States, most of them working for no compensation and providing close to $400 *billion* of free labor doing some of the most challenging jobs imaginable (Bastowrous (2013). In fact, it has been estimated that 90% of all long-term care needed by aging adults is assumed by unpaid family members or informal caregivers, almost all of whom are women (84%) and one-third of whom report significant stress (Adelman, Tmanova, Delgado, Dion, & Lachs, 2014). Although it has been found that such devotion provides an enriched life in some distinctive ways, there are also a number of severe stressors that leave caregivers suffering with their own problems (Box 9-1).

Family caregivers often feel a sense of helplessness watching their loved ones deteriorating, suffering in chronic pain, and barely functioning when completing the most rudimentary tasks. The elderly parent or spouse needs to be fed, bathed, and attended to on a constant basis. In some cases, these individuals have lost control of their bladder or bowels; in other cases of dementia, there can be unpredictable outbursts of rage or failure to recognize family members. And in many cases the caregivers rarely have the opportunity to tell their own stories and receive the support they need to continue their responsibilities. There has been precious few resources and help available to reduce their burden, and very little is understood by therapists about how to best intervene.

One of the main reasons for the burdens and stress associated with taking care of older family members is that the caregivers are untrained and inexperienced in the skills needed for this job. They often feel way over the heads because they receive so little support and preparation for their responsibilities. It is therefore suggested that, when therapists are assigned to cases with elderly clients who are

BOX 9-1 EFFECTS OF CAREGIVING WITH ELDERLY FAMILY MEMBERS

Burdens	**Gifts**
Sadness, grief, depression	Sense of purpose
Helplessness, anxiety	Increased self-esteem
Depletion of energy	Pride in accomplishment
Isolation and helplessness	Love and close attachment
Stigma and shame	Respect and merit in the community
Family conflicts	Family togetherness
Guilt and resentment	Fulfillment and gratitude
Financial pressures	New skills and knowledge
Self-neglect and fatigue	Expressions of love and gratitude

presenting severe medical conditions, they also assess the health and stress levels of their caregivers. This includes encouraging them to engage in their own self-care, as well as providing supplemental knowledge and information that may make their jobs easier.

Although the very term *caregiver* is associated with "burden," there are also many positive experiences that have been reported by those involved in this work. In addition to those "gifts" mentioned in Box 9-1, Mackenzie and Greenwood (2012) sought to identify more specifically what some of these enriching features might be for those most actively involved in taking care of elderly family members. This has important implications for our therapeutic strategies with these individuals because our focus can hone in on helping them to excavate and reframe these burdens as gifts. Examples of positive experiences that were reported most frequently included feeling (a) valued and appreciated, (b) increased self-worth, (c) better at coping with uncertainty, (d) clarity with regard to a future career path, (e) greater appreciation for life and every precious moment, (f) strengthened family relationships, (g) enjoyment of praise, and (h) mastery of skills related to medical or caretaking tasks. Knowledge of these common positive responses is important if our goal is to help such clients to balance their burdens and complaints with a greater appreciation for what they are learning and how they are growing as a result of their efforts.

Despite our best intentions to be supportive of caregivers, it is also not exactly uncommon that they will feel less than welcoming to our efforts. In some cases they may be downright hostile or obstructive, resenting our intrusions. In other cases their own mental health issues may be operating, and their sense of power and control may be threatened. As in other families in which there are dysfunctional dynamics going on, they may attempt actively to sabotage therapeutic efforts that appear to be in the best interests of the client. Agronin (2010) has characterized several types of the most challenging caregivers, including those who are suspicious, hostile, accusatory, and blaming; neglectful, passive–aggressive, and apathetic; overinvolved, hovering, and hypervigilant; and dependent and enmeshed. Before any attempt at systemic intervention, he recommends considering one's own personal reactions to the caregiver, asking oneself: How does this person make me feel? This can lead to some clues that help us to remain reasonably objective to be helpful not only to the client, but also to the family.

In one situation, an extremely dependent man in his 80s was kept closely under control by his much younger wife, who appeared to enjoy his total helplessness and dependence on her. Earlier in their relationship, before his stroke, he had been on the verge of divorcing her; now she actually seemed to enjoy the role reversal in which she held all the power. As such, any attempt by the physical therapist, occupational therapist, and speech therapist to teach the man a degree of self-sufficiency was actively compromised by the wife, who wanted her husband to remain helpless and dependent because of fears that he would otherwise leave her. Although this was not entirely possible because of the nature of his disabilities, it certainly made the therapist's job considerably more difficult because the wife was uncooperative and obstructive.

MAKING HOUSE CALLS

More and more often, therapists are providing in-home services, which have been found to produce a number of distinct advantages for those elderly people who are less mobile. This is an option that social workers have realized and responded to ever since the birth of their profession, yet now more and more mental health professionals are following this lead to conduct assessments, provide psychoeducational information, make appropriate referrals, and even conduct time-limited therapy sessions (Yang, Garis, Jackson, & McClure, 2009). This strategy allows elders to receive help who would otherwise be unable or unwilling to show up at a therapist's office, and it also helps the therapist to access a lot more information about a client's lifestyle, context, and situation. In addition, rapport is easier to establish and maintain, and there is much greater access to significant others who would play an important role in ongoing support and compliance with any treatment regimen.

Gerontological mental health specialists are as much life coaches as they are therapists in the roles and functions they serve. When working with older clients, traditional psychotherapy is often broadened to include attention to postretirement structure, social and economic realities, and lifestyle plans, and the sessions may take place in more nontraditional settings that include continual follow-up via phone, texts, video calls, or personal visits.

Of course there are challenges associated with doing therapy in a client's residence, including the high probability of distractions and interruptions. Boundaries are more difficult to establish and enforce. And a great deal of flexibility is required in the way sessions are conducted. If you have ever tried to lead a family therapy session with a large number of members present, then you can certainly appreciate the chaos and unpredictability that can arise, and how challenging it is to maintain a semblance of control. This is magnified many times when sitting in a client's residence when he or she keeps answering the phone, taking care of chores, talking to others in the house, or even falling asleep in a comfortable chair within a familiar environment.

And then there are the more complicated ethical issues that arise. How can confidentiality be enforced in a setting that has so much less privacy? How can informed consent be structured and explained? What about all the temptations for engaging in multiple relationships that are more likely in such a personal space? And what about the therapist's own safety, which not only includes working in areas that might be at greater risk for violence, but also being subjected to more volatile emotional reactions from the family, not to mention exposure to airborne diseases?

Yang et al. (2009) recommend minimizing these intrusive elements by planning for them ahead of time and instituting more structure than would normally be considered. These include (a) identifying one specific part of the house, including designated chairs, that are associated only with therapeutic work; (b) agreeing to a contract with strict rules for what will be discussed and what is considered off-limits (answering the phone, getting up to do chores, carrying on conversations with others who are around); (c) working more carefully on completing therapeutic tasks and assignments for which the client is held accountable; and (d) dealing directly with transference and countertransference issues considering the intimate setting in which sessions take place.

CHALLENGES OF OLDER THERAPISTS

We have been discussing throughout this book the ways that older therapists must make adjustments and adaptations in light of changes they experience in their own cognitive and physical functioning. This is no more apparent in the ways that time is treated differently. Claudia Black, a renowned addictions therapist, talked about the frustration she feels balancing time constraints.

"At this stage in life there is more of a reality that my time on this planet is limited, so this struggle is stronger for me now. I still feel passionate about my work but my personal life is very important too; I want time with family." Just as with our clients, this stage in life involves a number of additional challenges, such as taking care of parents as well as helping with adult children. And then there is the legacy of what you might wish to leave behind.

"At this age," Claudia admits, "I am more apt than someone younger to be thinking about what is on my headstone. Is it that I was great in my profession? No, not really. I hope I am good at what I do. I hope and believe I have made a contribution. I hope I help to make a difference in the lives of people and in this world."

Despite the pride of accomplishment she might feel, she also recognizes with humility that there are now many others to take her place. "When it is all said and done, there will always be other clinicians, therapists, leaders in our field, to continue my work, to make their own contributions." She is quick to point out, however, that although others may advance the professional work, there is nobody else to value her personal relationships.

Black also mentions another challenge that is commonly experienced by older people of every generation since the beginning of time—and that involves new advances in technology that make adjustments necessary. Just consider the number of people over 50 today who still can't program their digital recording devices on their televisions or even navigate the remote controls. Every few months there are updates to software on mobile phones, and every year the devices are reissued, rendering earlier models almost obsolete.

We remember a time when the only technology that had to be mastered in our profession was changing a typewriter ribbon or learning how to thread a movie projector (which wasn't all that easy!). Nowadays, a great deal of time and energy must be invested to remain even minimally current on state-of-the-art technology. Black mentions this as a hurdle in her own current practice.

"On a practical level, the integration of technology has been a challenge to my speaking career. Being in the addictions field, I facetiously say I had to complete a 'first step' once I surrendered to PowerPoint presentations versus the plastic transparencies I used to use."

Black mentions one other challenge that has required considerable adaptation, or perhaps acceptance of her current limitations. "Just the other day I was leading a group, and a part of the daily ritual in this residential program is choosing and then engaging in a yoga pose. Someone decided that we should all do 'the tree pose,' one of the simplest. I found myself with a group of 18- to 25-year-olds, all balanced on one leg, arms stretched high above heads. And let's just say I did not have the grace in balance they did."

Acceptance of realistic limits is a big part of dealing with the challenges. It helps that experience allows us to become more open to these inevitable physical changes. Black admits she is no longer intimidated by others as she once was, yet she also realizes that she sometimes feels out of touch with the experiences of her younger clients. She compensates for this, in part, by being more free to speak from the heart. "I have always enjoyed my work, and my passion is always strong.

But my passion only stays as strong as it is today with more time for my own self-care. I want time with my family and friends. I want time that includes wonderful outdoor exercise and recreation. I want time in Nature. Time is the big one."

Rosanne Tadsen was a school counselor for most of her life until a cascade of changes related to aging occurred that led to a career change. Her mother died recently, followed by her own diagnosis of a heart condition that led to a number of symptoms, including feeling unsteady and lightheaded. A few weeks ago she fell and broke her ankle.

"Fortunately," she related, "I was wearing a heart monitor that recorded the incident, and within several hours I had a pacemaker installed. None of that was on my to-do list that day. I am very definitely feeling mortal."

Tadsen retired from her job about six years ago and, because her entire existence had been "enriched by the energy and hope that comes from working with young people," she felt a mourning and loss that led her to search for something new and different. She decided to become credentialed as a licensed professional counselor and got a job in a counseling center, which she immediately noticed was quite different than working in a school—must more isolating and a *lot* quieter. A more striking difference, however, was how much more wisdom she brought to sessions than earlier in her career.

"As a younger counselor I was fascinated by the stories; as an older counselor I am honored that clients are willing to share their pain with me, and I am very much aware that their relief comes from their own strength and honesty. My having passed through some similar situations during my life only helps me understand the gravity of what I might not have understood when younger. It assists me in empathizing with my clients." She says this with a laugh because she admits to making a long list of mistakes in her life: "The older I become, the more I understand there is much that I don't understand!"

It has been a challenge to accept and get used to the idea that she is now an "elderly counselor." "It usually surprises and amuses me when a client makes reference to my elderly status. Several preteens, when telling a story about 'old people,' have paused in their story, looked a little embarrassed, and then said, 'Oh, I'm sorry!' "

Although several of her colleagues do treat her as a respected elder, other family members, friends, and peers wonder why she is still working at all. Why hasn't she moved to Florida with all the other "snowbirds" to play golf and bridge? "There seems to be an unwritten rule that there is a time to stop working, and not doing so throws the universe out of kilter. Even to Social Security, I am the 'working aged.' My carefully considered belief is that the gifts that I have been given as a human being are ageless, and I am supposed to keep using them in the best way that I can for as long as I can."

This particular attitude has served her well when working with elderly clients. "I have had the honor of counseling several older clients who were struggling with losses. They are honest, resilient people who were able to use the strength gleaned from a lifetime of success and disappointment to move on after losses that, at the time, seemed they would take over and end their lives. I have learned much about dignity and resilience by walking through sorrow with these clients."

As much as she enjoys her continued work, Tadsen admits she struggles with similar issues as her elderly clients, especially those who are facing challenges of intractable medical conditions. "My biggest challenge at this point is the awareness that life is finite and that I must prioritize carefully because I cannot do or have it all. My older clients have brought to me the concept of legacy and the idea that I can be intentional about the legacy I leave behind."

Tadsen has four grandchildren and she feels the most important work she is doing at this stage of life is really teaching them her most valuable life lessons. Her family is clearly her most important priority—a phenomenon that is actually age appropriate. She also spends a lot of time thinking about what she wishes to leave behind. "Today I visited the cemeteries where my parents and grandparents are buried and I had the opportunity to give their legacies some thought. I feel a bond with my ancestors that I have not felt before. I understand that I am not immortal and that, although there will be an increasing number of aspects of my life over which I will lose control, I need to understand what I still control and attend to it. I fear the loss of control that I know is in the future, as much from watching my mother struggle and react to it, as from seeing at as an inevitable but undefined part of what lies ahead."

JON: THE TIMES ARE CHANGING

I have noticed lately that I'm increasingly being asked questions I've never heard before. I was strolling along recently, my mind wandering, when my reverie was interrupted by an earnest young person who stopped and stared at me.

"Are you okay?" he asked.

I nodded my head, a little confused by the question. I looked down, checking out my body and wardrobe, wondering if there something wrong with me.

"Are you *sure* you're okay?" he asked once again. When I stared back at him, showing my annoyance, he walked on.

I wish I could say this was an anomaly, but more and more often since I entered "later maturity," people say things to me unprompted such as, "Do you need any help, Sir?" "Don't you have anyone to help you with that?" I feel like a helpless invalid at a time in my life when I should be reveling in my role as an honored sage. People used to ask me all the time, "So, what do you do?" Now they ask, "What is that you *used* to do?" I fear that soon the question will become instead, "What can you still do?"

I realize, of course, that I not only look old, but I am old, at least relative to many others around me. I also notice that I spend more and more time alone. My children and grandchildren have moved away to begin their own lives. Many of my oldest and dearest friends have retired or died. More and more often I'm being asked to write obituaries for lifelong colleagues; many others are ailing or failing.

I know that I am so fortunate to be still walking this earth, much less still doing therapy, teaching, and writing books. Given my cancer diagnosis it is a miracle of modern medicine that I am still alive, even with the various complications and lingering health problems that continue to plague me. I've had to learn to be dependent on others to take care of me. Clients and students seem to expect less of me, making allowances for my age, faltering memory, and "frail" condition. Just a few years ago I could run faster than anyone on the local high school cross-country team and now I seem just to shamble along.

Jon's awareness of the realities associated with aging, and especially how he is treated differently, presents one of the biggest challenges of all for older clients—and their therapists. People do expect less of them, and that also includes the more modest expectations that therapists have for what help their work can actually provide. We are certainly well aware that positive expectations, hope, and optimism are often associated with the best outcomes. And such an understanding has led our field to develop a number of specialized strategies and approaches that are ideally suited to maximize benefits for older clients.

PART IV

Journeys of Wisdom and Redemption

CHAPTER 10
Aging Is (Mostly) a State of Mind

How old would you be if you didn't know how old you was?

Satchel Paige, Baseball player

Earlier we discussed some of the myths associated with aging that have been perpetuated by media and other cultural scripts, leading to internalized self-perceptions that are quite limiting. This has encouraged many older people to feel they are doomed to loneliness, misery, disability, and despair. Yet, as we are certainly well aware, our beliefs and state of mind largely determine how people respond to the challenges they face in life, including those related to growing old. In fact, the more optimistic our views about the prospect of aging, and the more prepared we are for the likely realities, the better we can adapt to those challenges. Our job often involves helping older clients adopt more optimistic views of what is possible, an outcome that may actually reduce many of the negative effects of physical difficulties.

It's more than a little interesting that longevity may not be best predicted by genetic inheritance or even particular health markers such as blood pressure, cholesterol, weight, exercise, or smoking habits, but rather one's beliefs and attitudes about what it means to age. In one long-term study, people were asked what they think happens to them when they age (Levy et al., 2002). Those who thought that aging means you lose all your energy, become less useful and happy, and life generally becomes less satisfying, lived almost eight years less than those who thought otherwise!

RIGIDITY AND ITS CONSEQUENCES

There is little doubt that aging often brings with this maturity a tendency toward rigidity (Schafe, 2012). People become set in their ways, reluctant to change lifelong patterns, resistant to changes, even if they are no longer as functional as they had been in the past. This particular inflexible state of mind can compromise any progress that is made during therapy, as well as can lead to maladaptive attitudes that progress to chronic misery.

As cognitive therapy proponents have advocated for many years, people are perfectly capable of learning to think differently about their life challenges and stress levels, especially during high emotional arousal. In the words of William James, "the greatest weapon against stress is our ability to choose one thought over another."

In one representative study, participants were taught to monitor their physiological arousal such as heartbeat, breathing, and other responses during a stressful situation. The researchers found that such a strategy helped them to develop more adaptive and moderate responses that included increased cardiovascular efficiency that accompanied more measured thought processes (Jamieson, Nock, & Mendes, 2012). It was truly an example of mind over matter.

In another, far different example of how perceptions and beliefs affect health and aging, Keller et al. (2012) found that if you believe that stress will affect your health significantly and profoundly, then it will indeed do so at a greater level than might otherwise occur. Those who believe that stress affected their health a lot increased their risk of premature death by as much as 43%! This leads us to challenge some of the entrenched or erroneous beliefs that older clients bring to sessions, such as the ideas that aging means they must necessarily reduce all stress and new challenges to preserve their continued health or avoid significant disability. Resilience and heartiness are key resources that help older people deal with adjustments, feel a greater sense of control, and handle adversity better (Seery, Holman, & Silver, 2010). This is one of the premises of the posttraumatic growth movement—that what doesn't kill you can potentially make you stronger if you are able to metabolize the experience in a more constructive way (Calhoun & Tedeschi, 2013; Joseph, 2011; Neimeyer, 2004).

Rigid cognitive patterns that have become grooved during a lifetime of experience are quite difficult to alter because of neurological pathways in the brain that result from habitual responses (Duhigg, 2012). The consequences of this process that saves time and energy is that future options may be limited. Indeed, the sort of rigid thinking that may be characteristic of older clients limits their ability—and willingness—to consider multiple ways of looking at their predicament and developing alternative solutions to the problems.

Strategic and brief therapists such as Jay Haley, Cloe Madanes, Bill O'Hanlon, Steve de Shazer, Insoo Kim Berg, and others observed a long time ago that when people feel stuck in helpless situations, it is often because they keep doing the same things over and over, although it is clear the approach is not working. One older couple in their 70s who had ongoing conflict in their relationship kept engaging in the same circular causality that is so common in systemic dysfunction. Marilyn, the wife, kept nagging her husband, Jake, to stick with a diet to prevent additional heart disease. He so resented the controlling, scolding tone, that he would deliberately eat forbidden foods, not so much because he craved them as because he knew it annoyed his wife. When it was pointed out to Marilyn that her nagging wasn't producing the outcome she (and the doctors) desired, she felt helpless to stop doing what was already not working. Until such time that she could break this habit, she was unable to experiment with other strategies that might be more effective. Jake just found all of this quite amusing and seemed to enjoy the power he wielded, pushing his wife's buttons by hiding Snickers bars around the house.

Quite another kind of flexibility and adaptation is evident in Hank's situation. He is a lawyer and municipal judge in his 70s. He suffered a second nearly fatal heart attack 20 years earlier. He had actually been clinically dead and had to be "paddled" back to consciousness. This got his attention in ways nothing had earlier, launching him in the direction of becoming a marathon runner that he believed would literally save his life and disrupt his previously poor lifestyle habits of sloth and gluttony.

Hank also decided to reinvent himself in other ways, deciding that 50 was really not too old to start over. He went back to graduate school to become a therapist, even though it took him eight years to complete the training because of his legal responsibilities, heart transplant, cancer diagnosis, and surgeries. And yet, when all was said and done, he had never been happier and more satisfied.

"It isn't cancer or heart disease that will always kill you," Hank said with a laugh, "it's retirement!" Hank found that disengaging from everything he once loved left him feeling lost, and he desperately needed goals to shoot for, whether improving his marathon times or making a difference in his community not only as a compassionate judge, but also as a counselor.

Hank also observed other ways his change in attitude and state of mind has made it possible for him to adjust to aging in ways he hadn't expected. Applying his newfound counseling skills to himself certainly helped, as did the encouragement of family and friends, to stay hopeful and positive.

BEING CAUTIOUS AND CONSERVATIVE

Any political election would confirm that older people tend to be more conservative and cautious than those who are younger. This would be equally true with respect to managing finances. Such a perspective is sometimes highly adaptive in that the risk–reward outcomes are different for those who don't have the time, resources, or energy to recover from a misjudgment. This is by no means the same thing as being stubborn or rigid, which does often stem from maladaptive attitudes.

During one family session attended by a couple and the father's 86-year-old mother, they complained about a recent family reunion attended by all the grandchildren. Before the kids even arrived to the house for the event, the grandmother decided to return to her own apartment because it was the only place she felt comfortable using the bathroom. This wasn't about safety issues, because the couple had installed rails near their own toilet specifically for this purpose; it was related to the grandmother's habitual fears. Because of that behavior, she missed seeing her grandchildren, who returned to college after the party was over.

What we often do for a living is to challenge such cautious and conservative attitudes that get in the way of more fully functioning options. Whether inclined toward a therapeutic approach that is cognitive–behavioral, narrative, feminist, psychodynamic, relational–cultural, emotionally focused, or any other, all of us push clients to examine more carefully and critically their beliefs and assumptions that are self-liming. Of course it is one thing to talk about this in sessions and quite another to encourage older clients to put these ideas into practice on a daily basis. Hill (2005) suggests direct efforts to address this problem by encouraging, recommending, prescribing older clients to get outside their comfort zones deliberately to try new options that might limber them up to increase their willingness and flexibility to make other needed changes. This could include such things as the following:

- Take a different route to familiar places.
- Approach a stranger to start a conversation.
- Predict how you might typically respond to someone—and instead say something new or different.
- Take a different political position on a social issue in a conversation, just to present an alternative point of view.
- Literally get dressed in the morning in a varied sequence—put on socks *before* underwear or brush teeth *after* brushing hair—anything to change routines.
- Order a different food or meal in a restaurant instead of what you usually select.
- Keep a daily journal of everything you tried for the first time.

One other way that cautious and conservative attitudes are problematic is when they lead to consistently negative or pessimistic thinking. We might hear statements like, "This just isn't like the good ol' days" or "It'll probably never work anyway" or "What's the use?" This kind of belief system has its own benefits in that it protects people from disappointment, especially for those who have already suffered so much in their lives; they've learned to expect very little and to anticipate the worst. They also get to blame others when things inevitably go wrong. In some ways, they can even enjoy a feeling of control in that they don't get their hopes dashed. But this also comes at a cost in that all their needless worry leads to chronic discouragement and unhappiness, even if this takes place on their own terms.

METABOLIZING TRAUMA THROUGHOUT LIFE

One of the most interesting—and perplexing—phenomena related to ways people deal with life challenges is how their memories of those events and crises evolve as they age. In some cases, difficult and traumatic events lose their

JEFFREY: KEEPING PAINFUL MEMORIES ALIVE

I have had a few clients who took their lives during the time I was seeing them, and this led to major crises of despair, discouragement, and self-recrimination. I reasoned that if only I was smarter, better trained, more perceptive, more vigilant, I could have somehow prevented these tragedies. Supervision afterward, as well as years of self-reflection, helped me to realize I really had done all I could. Despite my yearning for perfectionism, I accept my limitations and inability to control and predict the future. Over time, I have become much more forgiving of failures that were not really within my power to control completely. Occasionally, I am still haunted by the ghosts of those I couldn't reach—or save—but I have learned to let the memories go, and they have indeed faded over time. I attribute this to the maturity and experience that comes with age.

On the other hand . . . yes, you can sense what is coming. My true confession is that there are a few cases in which, rather than losing their power to haunt me, I have allowed them to blossom and grow way out of proportion to their actual meaning at the time. Most of these relate to interpersonal conflicts with colleagues. I remember one colleague who, let's just say, had very different notions about professionalism. I would say, in retrospect, he was one of the most rigid, judgmental people I've ever known. But another interpretation is that he just had my number and I was found wanting in his eyes. There was nothing I could do to satisfy his standards, many of which didn't jibe with my own. I have worked in therapy, supervision, journaling, and so much self-talk to purge this guy out of my head. I never liked him. I never respected him. Most of the time I didn't agree with him about hardly anything. But his power to disturb me has actually grown throughout the years. Of course the feelings of critical judgment from him come in waves—there might be months that go by that I don't think about him—but then at the most surprising and inopportune moments, especially when I'm trying to fall asleep, I see him shaking his head at me and giving that scornful look.

I know this doesn't exactly qualify as "trauma," but more of an annoying memory from the past, but I have allowed this virus to flourish as I age. The therapist in me would say I need this memory, that I keep it as a warning or a punishment or perhaps an object lesson. And I suppose over time I have learned to live it, just as we all keep painful events alive.

power over time; in other cases, they seem to grow in magnitude like a virus out of control.

Whether in the role of therapists, or in everyday life, all of us have compartmentalized painful events, relegated them to long-term storage in some obscure warehouse of our memory, or else kept them very much front and present, as is typical of reoccurring trauma and ongoing stress. We might even expect that the longer we live, the more such trauma and suffering will bubble to the surface.

In studies of those who have lived more than a century, there is every reason to expect they would not only be enfeebled, but also most vulnerable to stress. After all, they've likely not only lost their spouse and all their friends, as well as possibly their children, but practically everything else that was ever familiar to them. Their health would be precarious—pain, a constant companion. They may have limited financial means and be stored in a residential facility. In other words, we'd have every reason to expect that centenarians would be the most depressed, alienated, and anxious people around. So it is surprising that most of them are hardly traumatized, and most of them are quite happy and content with their lives, however limited they may appear to others. It is surmised that one reason for their relatively optimistic, adaptive condition is that, in every sense of the word, they are truly survivors (Martin, Da Rosa, & Poon, 2011). Any trauma from past episodes has long been put behind them. Their expectations are modest; just waking up in the morning, even with all the aches and infirmities, is a wonderful gift. As a function of achieving the ripe old age of 100, they enjoy special status and feel heroic in this endeavor. They are also obviously high in characteristics such as resilience and robustness. They seem to have developed an immunity to little things that might be unduly disturbing to others who perished long ago.

SUBJECTIVE EXPERIENCE OF DAILY LIFE

There have actually been surprisingly few studies investigating how older people think about and experience their daily lives. In one of the few studies exploring lifestyle issues, the main themes identified were associated with coming to terms with existential issues related to the meaning of life—and of death (Borglin, Edberg, & Hallberg, 2005). Just as we have been discussing, researchers discovered that successful adjustment to aging was a subjective experience rather than the way things might appear to others. Among the people in their 80s who they interviewed, one of the most consistent findings was how important it was to have developed a reasonably coherent, meaningful "life course"—to be able to tell one's story in such a way that it felt connected to the present. In fact, living in the present was considered one of the single most important facets of a positive adjustment to being old, taking each day as a gift, maintaining a sense of wonder rather than brooding about the past. Those who enjoyed their life the most took pleasure from their daily activities—going for walks, meeting friends, spending time with family, shopping, exercising, reading, playing cards. It was critical that each day had meaning, rather than worrying unduly about an uncertain future.

It seemed especially important to these oldsters in their 80s that they had the opportunity to share their life stories with others, that somehow there was special meaning in what they had witnessed and lived throughout their presence in the world. This is where and how therapy can be so incredibly useful to almost anyone at this age. People need to tell their stories. They need to make sense of what they lived. They need to shape the narratives in such a way that they become heroes of their own journey. And they need to talk about this to others in such a way that their life experiences meant something to themselves and others.

Leita, mentioned earlier, believes that attitude is everything in coming to terms with the challenges she faces. She prefers to focus on the gifts she receives every day rather than the obstacles she encounters. And with a husband who is dying of cancer, she faces more than her fair share.

"I appreciate and love my husband more than ever. My love for him feels more passionate, even though our physical sex life is gone. I also love my family more and seem to judge them less." She reports that becoming a grandmother helped her with this, but also her commitment to social causes. "I feel very lucky that I lived during the vibrant years of scientific and political revolution, and was a small part of these movements. When I am having a good day, I feel proud of the work I did over the years."

Although Leita speaks of these days of activism as if they are long over, she is still quite involved in environmental causes, both within her local community and on a larger scale. She refuses to own a car or travel by plane, which she considers abusive of the environment. She became involved in political elections.

Her positive state of mind has also helped her to let go of resentments in the past. "Time passes and there is healing. I am so appreciative of my good fortune to have a good family, a wonderful husband, a nice place to live. I can still walk and cycle, take care of my husband, and still have a couple shots of Tequila without having to finish the bottle."

It is also important that she retains a professional identity. "My dad used to say that he never got much respect as an artist in his professional life, but he never ran out of things to do. This is one of the blessings of being a painter in that I can still see, draw, and paint, and have a good time doing it."

STORYTELLING IN LATER LIFE

It is another one of the myths about aging that older people may subscribe to the idea that the stories of their life are almost over. This is what Freeman (2011)

JON: BEING OLD AND FEELING USELESS

Aging has impacted my hearing, seeing, walking, driving, thinking, and memory, and it gets me wondering every morning when I wake up: What's next? I feel a declining usefulness, almost a sense of incompetence, even after devoting a lifetime to becoming really, really good at what I do. For the first time in my life, I have a fear of failure. I wonder if I should keep all these fears and concerns to myself and pretend I don't notice the ways people treat me differently.

It would be logical to diagnose myself as depressed. After all, sex has certainly changed, just as I notice I'm not touched as often. I feel a distance between myself and others, or at least imagine this is the case. I think of all the movies I've seen with creepy old codgers. I picture children shrinking away from me in fear. I worry that, rather than being seen as wise, I am becoming a foolish old man.

It doesn't seem so long ago that I had an unlimited future. Now everything seems limited to me. I realize I don't have that much longer to live, a finite, a countable number, of years—perhaps even days. I notice that my reasons for living have changed accordingly in ways that sometimes parallel what I see in my older clients. I hear them talk about their fears of ending up in a nursing home, sick and alone. I used to listen to these stories and shake my head at what struck me as a gross, exaggerated fantasy; now I wonder if that is where I will end up.

I have second thoughts about revealing all these concerns. It feels taboo to talk about them. I know that little of this was ever part of my training and preparation as a therapist. Sure, there are gerontology classes these days, but I've encountered relatively little about working clinically with the aged, and especially so when the therapist, too, is considered elderly or even middle-aged. There seems to be so much to know and learn and understand, especially with regard to the changes that each of us is living through.

has called "narrative foreclosure," in which people think they are just running out the course of their life with nothing much new to add to the story. He thinks this is not only wrong, but also is the primary reason for existential despair that may strike during this time. It is therefore our job to keep the life story open and unfolding, to review what has happened until this point, and be supportive of adding new chapters as well.

Storytelling is, in fact, the way we construct and make sense of the world, as well as connect to others, among their other functions (Gottschall, 2012; Kottler, 2015) that are listed here.

- It is through stories that older people pass along wisdom and knowledge to others in the community, providing critical information that increases the likelihood of continued survival. Traditionally, this meant sharing stories about hunting grounds, battles, births, deaths, and traditions, but it can also include any valuable information about past mistakes, failures, and triumphs.
- Throughout human history there has been power and status afforded to the most accomplished storytellers, who served important roles as entertainers and teachers. The job of elders was to tell the stories of the past as a way to acculturate young people into the traditions, rituals, and history of the tribe. Even today, successful screenwriters, novelists, actors, and media celebrities are compensated extraordinarily well for the functions they serve.
- Stories provide a kind of vicarious experience for listeners, readers, and viewers, all without putting themselves in jeopardy or risk. That is one reason why murder mysteries, zombie films, serial killer novels, and violent shows are so popular; they allow people to imagine themselves in life-threatening situations and work through how they might survive such trials. Older people also have a responsibility to pass along those seminal stories of their life that resulted in potential risks for others.
- It is through stories that any group becomes bonded together. The reminiscing that is common among older people isn't just about honoring past achievements and joys, but about reminding families and groups about their shared connections. Any story that begins with, "Remember the time when . . . ," is really about strengthening tribal connections.
- Stories assist people in the integration of losses and trauma. Memories and intrusive negative experiences from the past must be processed in such a way that they are incorporated into a coherent narrative. Whether shared with family members, friends, or a therapist, older people need opportunities to talk about their life difficulties and work through them.
- Almost all life experiences that stay with us are processed into storied memories. Dreams and fantasies are remembered only when these fragments are converted into stories. Two-thirds of all conversations that people have with one another involve telling stories about oneself or others. Even most of our own most memorable training experiences involved hearing case examples or stories that held within them important lessons.

In one sense, what therapists do for a living is honor people's stories and tell other stories that are intended to impact and influence people (Kottler, 2015). Whether in the form of self-disclosures, metaphors, parables, illustrative examples, or teaching tales, we often spend our time with clients exchanging stories with one another.

An older client told one version of a story in which she felt stuck and without many choices. She felt dependent on others, helpless, and without hope. And then we introduced another possible version of the way this story could be configured, one that offered a different future and certainly a modified present that focused on opportunities, options, and possibilities that hadn't been considered before.

WHEN THE MIND CREATES NEW MEANING

Although this emphasis on storytelling and meaning-making is certainly the priority of narrative and constructivist therapies, we believe all therapists use these strategies in their work, and never more so than with aging clients. Nothing we do is more important that listening to and honoring their life stories, and helping them to shape them in ways that emphasize their strengths and resources. The stories they share reveal the most positive and trying times of their lives, especially in the very old and those suffering from dementia (Bruce, 1999), but also any clients who want to make sense of their lives (Bergner, 2007; Burns, 2007; Ingemark, 2013; Kottler, 2015; Mehl-Madrona, 2010).

A whole new field of narrative gerontology (Kenyon, Bohlmeijer, & Randall, 2011) and narrative medicine emphasizes the importance of physicians and health professionals listening to their patients' stories of illness and suffering, instead of only seeking a medical or surgical solution to a problem (Charon, 2001, 2006; Mehl-Madrona, 2007). As we mentioned earlier, this is especially important given that patients are rarely allowed to finish their stories or feel understood by their doctors (Levine, 2004).

We know from all kinds of advancements during the past few years that the stories people tell themselves about their lives become the reality of what (they believe) actually occurred. Experiences of isolation, for instance, are based on interpretations of one's life as much as any daily social engagement, often related to expectations. It is a reality that people interact with fewer people as they age, but that doesn't necessarily mean the relationships are any less satisfying. Those in study by Borglin et al. (2005) who reported having the most meaningful life felt included rather than left out of family and social interactions, but this was based on their perceptions of what was appropriate contact. The quality of their lives was improved significantly when they were offered opportunities to contribute to the conversation in some way and to feel valued for what they offered.

For those who don't feel like they have such consistent opportunities, therapy offers the perfect place to have one. It is important to older people that they not feel like a nuisance to others, which is why it is often so helpful to be able to talk to therapists and other health professionals to take up some of the slack without feeling like they are burdensome. Of course this means the therapist's own attitudes, and state of mind, should communicate to older clients that they are honored and valued.

Successful treatment of aging clients is clearly based on the therapist's welcoming presence. Although they are speaking specifically about their interpersonal therapy model for elderly depression, Hinrichsen and Clougherty (2006) mention several impediments to successful outcomes. The first and foremost problem is the therapist's own belief that not much can be accomplished in a relatively short period of time. If you think an older client's issues are permanent, chronic, intractable, and impervious to change, then whatever follows is going to be less effective than would otherwise be possible with a more optimistic, hopeful prognosis.

Let's face it: the best predictor of adjustment to aging isn't so much one's health, but rather one's socioeconomic resources. In addition, in studies of the "oldest old" (85+ years), well-being is usually determined by social support, spiritual affiliation, leisure pursuits, nutrition, personality traits such as hardiness, and the "will to live" (Poon & Cohen-Mansfield, 2011). Religious and spiritual matters become much more important to the elderly as they approach the prospect of death and search for integrative meaning in their life (Fry, 2000; Oritz & Langer, 2002). Such existential matters become an important focus of therapy and often become the center of therapeutic work, whether in explorations of a Higher Power, Nature, wonder and awe, or the essence of Self (Suri, 2010).

Writing about the search for meaning in later life, MacKinlay (2014) concludes that life satisfaction is not really related to financial resources (within reason), nor is it connected to good health, but rather to the attitude one has adopted to face any age-related challenges. Any cognitive, narrative, or existential therapist places at its core the creation of meaning in experience.

"Why is it," she asks, "that some older people, despite disabilities and chronic disease, find peace and joy, while others seem to be in a state of despair?" (MacKinlay, 2014, p. 114). The answer, she suggests, is found as the elderly enter a kind of "natural monastery," where there are opportunities for greater contemplation, introspection, and meaning-making. This is what helps people to transcend pain, fear, and discomfort. And it is our job to help older clients reach a state of self- transcendence where they can seek forgiveness and emphasize gratitude, as well as keep a sense of humor. It also helps if we model such attitudes in our own characteristic ways of being.

Catherine, a 70-year-old therapist born in the final days of the Second World War, remembers the deprivations she experienced as a child with limited food and staples available. "I remember being horrified when viewing the photographs of Holocaust survivors in *Life Magazine* and telling my preschool self that if I had just been born a few years earlier I could have saved them. I remember the school drills for nuclear war when, confused, I wondered if I would ever see my family again. I remember law, business, and medical schools that had a quota of two to four women admitted for every 100 men. And now I remember people who once inhabited my life and they are now gone—my parents, grandparents, a sibling, beloved friends, and mentors who shaped me personally and professionally."

Catherine paused for a moment of silent reflection and then declared that all these people are still alive through her, and this gets her wondering how she will be kept alive after she is gone. "I know I will die and that it won't likely be decades from now. I find myself hoping it won't be decades from now; this could mean years of disability and running out of savings."

Catherine adjusted her work as a therapist considerably when she began to specialize in older clients, mostly men, in later life. "They appear in my office, shattered by events largely beyond their control: the spouse who abruptly left for a new partner with little explanation; the wife whose husband, diagnosed with cognitive impairment, no longer remembers much of their history together and will need continuing care; the "empty nesters" who can no longer find meaning or pleasure in their relationship; the financial debacle of a business venture that has stolen critical retirement savings; the man who has always lived the much-touted healthy life stricken with aggressive lung cancer despite never having smoked."

Such issues have encouraged Catherine to become a "midwife" to help create new meanings and states of mind. She finds that one reason she can be so persuasive and effective is because she shares many of the same fears and challenges as so many of her older clients. She sees her job these days as helping people "to find joy hiding in full sight, even in the sorrows."

Catherine finds it a great advantage to already "know" her older clients as they have shared so much with her. "While care and attention need to be given to the therapeutic alliance and to developing a way of being together, we are already partway there. We know that with effort, disappointments in the work we do together can be healed. In the faces of each other, in our eyes, we see a person who has lived awhile, who is bound to have suffered loss, imperfection, confusion, regret—these experiences that tell us we are in only partial control of our lives."

She has observed such feelings of shame in her older clients because they feel so much like a burden or have lost their sense of control. She has more therapeutic leverage than ever before because her clients recognize that the time left is so limited and precious. And yet she has found they are able to relax and let go, "to take off the masks we wear, to express the true depth of despair, and even to laugh ruefully about what is before us, though in this case it is the client's story. We are in this together, which is always true, but sometimes denied."

Catherine has found that with her older clients they expect a certain expertise, but they also don't want her sitting on some "high throne of knowledge." It is far more important to be fully, authentically present with them. "Older clients have learned that there aren't easy 'fixes,' even as they might also wish for the magic wand of transformation. Distress and suffering are hard and exhausting. It's in our nature to want to escape them while still finding meaning in the difficult journey through and beyond them."

What comes through so loud and clear in Catherine's words is the pure joy she feels being in the company of her older clients. She loves the freedom that she can give up the role of being a "know-it-all" and instead share with them the "songs of living," being less defined "by what we do, by the age of our bodies, than by how we choose to live." She ended her thoughts by asking a singularly important question that is all about promoting hope: "What if we couldn't wait to be an older person to enjoy these delicious fruits of an honestly lived life?"

PROMOTING HOPE

So much of our job involves selling hope to those who feel discouragement and despair. This is true regardless of the age and stage in life. An adolescent girl with an eating disorder told her therapist she is doomed and that her life is essentially over because of the bridges she has already burned; we help her to envision a quite different future within her grasp. A father went to therapy feeling completely incompetent as a parent because his five-year-old son acts out in preschool, just as he did when he was that age, and we present an alternative perspective, and guidance, that leads in a far more optimistic direction. And a woman in her 60s, who just lost her husband to a sudden stroke, believed her life was over and she would never find anything resembling happiness and satisfaction again. The therapist persuades her to be patient during her period of grief and readjustment, and helps her to see little reasons, already, why her future is not so dismal as she imagines. In each of these cases, and so many others, our work begins with promoting a more optimistic, hopeful picture of what could be possible.

There is a connection between the sort of posttraumatic growth that sometimes occurs after a crisis or tragedy and what happens during advanced aging, when people face difficult health issues and adjustments that may lead to greater wisdom and well-being. Similar to posttraumatic growth after recovering from a trauma, change is promoted through a shattering loss that triggers existential reflection. This has been described as *gerotranscendence,* a condition in which challenges in later life lead to dramatic alterations in the perception of oneself, others, and the larger world (Tornstam, 2005). The losses can often facilitate new insights that disrupt the status quo and lead to greater appreciation for the most ordinary events. Both forms of adjustment to loss facilitate deeper exploration of essential questions of meaning: "Who am I now?" and "What am I here for?"

Weiss (2014) summarizes the mechanisms and stages of gerotranscendence as following processes we would also recognize in clients who are experiencing growth after recovering from any life difficulty or challenge:

1. There is a disruption of usual, familiar, and ordinary daily routines, often in the form of a catastrophic loss.
2. This results in disorientation, confusion, and struggle.
3. Constructive rumination and reflection may result in alternative ways of viewing options.
4. Explorations of meaning and purpose widen further the scope of possibilities.
5. There may often be an enhanced spiritual worldview.
6. A more robust and altered form of self-transcendence results from such deep explorations, and challenges of the status quo and what must be.
7. There is a shift in corresponding life priorities and values.
8. Losses are reframed as opportunities for new possibilities.
9. Increased wisdom and life satisfaction are the accumulative gifts of such a process.

Just as the case with most any trauma, a significant number of people—estimated at roughly one-third—are able to recover from the incident, not only regaining their previous level of functioning without lingering symptoms, but also experiencing dramatic and life-altering personal transformations for which they feel grateful (Calhoun & Tedeschi, 2013; Joseph, 2011). That, after all, is one of our primary tasks: to help our clients of whatever age to envision who they are, who they might become, and what might be possible.

CHAPTER 11

Specialized Strategies for Working with Older Clients

He who is of a calm and happy nature will hardly feel the pressure of age, but to him who is of an opposite disposition, youth and age are equally a burden.

Plato

As we covered previously, historically there has been a marked reluctance on the part of therapists to work with older clients, believing many are too old to change and too rigid in their thinking to respond well to treatment. It was actually several of Freud's disciples such as Carl Jung, Hannah Segal, and Alfred Adler who were far more optimistic and interested in extending the theory in ways that would be applicable to later life. Karl Abraham (1919), in particular, was instrumental in developing treatment strategies to be more responsive to his older clients, noting these were actually some of his most successful cases. He didn't care much about how old his clients were; rather, he was a lot more concerned with the age in which their problems developed.

Contrary to the prevailing attitudes of many psychodynamic therapists during the early years, Plotkin (2014) and many others have found that older adults are often ideal for extended therapy. Because aging is associated with more life experience, greater emotional control, better patience, longer periods of critical reflection, and dedicated motivation to meaning-making, in some ways the elderly are ideal candidates for insight-oriented explorations. Of course such therapeutic relationships are not without special challenges, which we have mentioned before, especially those related to potential memory loss, entrenched patterns, and physical limitations.

There have been several significant changes that have now created a completely new landscape for this specialty of working with older clients. First of all, life expectancy has increased dramatically, as have advances in medicine to prolong life. These changes have created a corresponding demand for therapeutic services—and where there is a market share to fill, there is always an opportunity for new enterprises. As the healthcare system becomes increasingly integrated and inclusive, there are also more ways that mental health professionals' expertise is in demand. New research on cognitive changes during aging support the idea that old dogs really can learn new tricks, providing a greater incentive for developing new, adaptive models of intervention. Challenges to ageism and biases against older people also create a more supportive climate. In addition, the goals of therapy have expanded considerably in recent years, just as specialized strategies for working with this population have evolved as well.

This chapter is longer than the others in this book because there is so much territory to cover related to the specialized approaches and strategies that have been customized for older clients. Because training in this specialty is becoming increasingly popular as a result of the increasing number of older clients who seek therapeutic services, we recommend that you consult some of the major sources mentioned in the pages that follow.

ADAPTING POPULAR MODELS TO A DIFFERENT KIND OF CLIENT

Let's begin with a reminder that the vast majority of therapeutic approaches were not designed for older adults, nor have they been adapted significantly to work with this population in the same ways that there has been such an emphasis on sensitivity to gender, ethnicity, religion, and other cultural factors. For so many years, many of the major theorists believed that the elderly were lost causes with respect to making major life changes because it was believed they were too rigid and stubborn.

Alfred Adler was one notable exception to the early psychodynamic theorists who focused their efforts almost exclusively on the young and middle-aged. "Not much is done for old people in our culture," Adler observed, noting that they appear to feel "futile and useless" (as cited in Ansbacher & Ansbacher, 1956, p. 43), trying to prove their worth and value just as they did during adolescence. He believed that one main problem is that they so often feel overlooked and disappointed

Although Adler did not write much about working with the elderly some of his ideas have been adapted easily for use with this population. For instance, Ionedes (1992), a psychiatrist who used an Adlerian-based approach for working with Alzheimer's disease, framed the illness as far more than just an individual problem. Effective treatment requires the involvement of the patient's immediate family, the network of key relatives and friends, and the elements of the larger social community. He used medication, individual and group psychotherapy (including psychodrama), and even social events such as dance parties. Ionedes (1979) would hold regular parties at his home, where 50 to 100 people would attend. Half would be mental patients and the other half would be his relatives, friends, and neighbors. At these gatherings, his patients would learn social skills, etiquette, and a variety of popular dance methods.

Solis and Brink (1992) highlight some other ways Adler's ideas have been adapted for older clients. They discuss how to work with the "Four Ds" that account for most of the mental problems of the elderly: delirium, dementia, depression, and delusional disorders. They describe the importance of being flexible in finding unique strategies to serve elderly clients, especially when most manuals fail to adapt procedures to age-specific contexts. Sperry (1992) described the legacy of how Adlerian ideas can be integrated easily with the treatment perspectives of cognitive–behavioral, experiential, psychodynamic, and systems approaches when working with older adults. Duffy (1992), as well, looked at some of the specific applications of Adlerian work to some elderly problems related to marital disruption and eating problems. Sperry (1992) also describes how Adlerian ideas can be used with adult children of aging parents. And more broadly, O'Connell (1992) viewed Adler's ideas as having the basic ingredients for a most productive "elderhood." One of his most creative ideas was the establishment of encouragement volunteers. These are people who were trained to visit the elderly, spreading encouragement and positive thoughts.

PARALLEL PROCESSES

Although this chapter title refers to "strategies" for working with older clients, and indeed there are a few specialized approaches that are optimal for this population, we have seen how many of the adjustments we make involve our own internal attitudes. Therapists are known to avoid working with the elderly, or make distorted or biased judgments, largely because of the ways we feel stuck within their own emotional reactions. Kraus (2012) warns about the emotional risks involved in this work, triggering terror of the therapist's own vulnerability, dependency, and existential crises. It is not just the prospect of physical death that comes with the territory, but also cognitive death that can result from dementia and profound memory loss.

Although Kraus feels true joy in working with older clients, he well understands the reluctance that many others feel to get involved because of the perceived risks. Yet, when misguided assumptions are challenged—that the elderly can't benefit much from therapy or that they are too rigid and stubborn to change—there are wonderful new growth opportunities for both therapists and their clients to face parts of themselves that have been disowned or ignored. "This has been part of my joy in working with older clients," Kraus admits. "I am able to honor them, to sit at their feet, marvel, and learn. As their therapist, I have become their faithful student, their privileged witness, and my life is ever richer because of it" (Kraus, 2012).

Maude and William had been in therapy for almost 20 years, beginning when they were in their late 50s. William was a large, overweight man who was self-centered and abusive whereas Maude was diminutive and appeared mousey and timid. Long before Maude began the sessions, she had been dealing with an aggressive respiratory problem that was potentially life-threatening; she was only given a few years left before the disease might very well kill her.

Since she received this diagnosis, Maude had tried to find, and then to keep, her voice—meaning, she needed, finally, to stand up to William and his bullying. During the early stages of treatment there was much miscommunication, anger, threats, tears, and emotion that filled the consulting room. As time went on, Maude decided to divorce her abusive husband and asked that he leave their home. Their three adult children tried to remain connected to each parent, but they also struggled with their own issues. The eldest daughter had an eating disorder, the middle daughter was in treatment for heroin addiction, and the youngest son could not hold a job and had great hatred for the way his father treated his mother. The family was a mess.

Throughout the 20 years of treatment, the couple lived in separate residences. The kids left home and began families of their own. Maude continued to have breathing problems but developed a fierce determination to stand up to William whenever he was around. He stopped by her house several days each week to take care of her and to clean the house, cook meals, and to wait on her as she did him when they had first met. The difference was that he was now acting out of love and devotion, rather than a position of dominance and control. Eventually, through a long and patient journey, they learned to love one another and negotiate a truce. Their only regret was that they had waited into their later years to take steps they wished they had taken so many years earlier.

Their therapist, as well, found that, during this prolonged and sometimes agonizing collaboration that spanned two decades, he had been forced to deal with some unresolved issues of his own that had been playing out in his marriage and with one of his own children.

"Each time I see this resilient couple," he commented, "I am so impressed with their courage and resilience to put death on hold while they faced the business of living their lives."

CUSTOMIZED STRATEGIES FOR OLDER CLIENTS

There have been therapeutic approaches designed specifically for older clients, beginning the work of Martin (1944) and Hildebrand (1990), as well as strategies summarized by Hepple (2004); Knight (2004); Dening and Thomas (2013); Frazer, Hinrichsen, and Jongsma (2014); and others. Many of the manualized treatments tend to be rather specifically focused on symptomatic relief and management of presenting complaints without much concern for relational issues or a search for deeper meaning. For instance, an older person presenting with depression kicks in a treatment plan that follows a series of sequential steps: (a) identify specific symptoms of depression, as well as their precipitating factors, situations, and context; (b) administer a geriatric depression scale; (c) identify primary components of the depression; (d) conduct a medical assessment and review of medications; (e) instruct client to keep a daily chart of mood ratings; (f) challenge unrealistic and dysfunctional thinking; (g) compile a list of common self-defeating thoughts; (h) assign homework to engage in positive self-talk; (i) assess daily activities that are viewed most pleasant and unpleasant; (j) discuss lifestyle changes that would be most advantageous; (k) construct a weekly schedule that includes more desirable activities; (l) teach warning signs of recurrence of symptoms, and (m) measure outcome.

Obviously, such a treatment plan is heavily steeped in cognitive–behavioral and behavioral strategies, many of which may indeed be useful. Nevertheless, so many of the concerns that older clients bring to therapy don't necessarily lend themselves to mere symptomatic improvement; they also involve the strong desire to be heard, understood, valued, respected, to feel connected, to discover meaning and purpose in a life lived well, and, most importantly, to feel a commitment to make the most of whatever time is left.

Nevertheless, when a specific therapeutic modality such as cognitive therapy is used when treating older adults it must be adapted and customized just as we would with any particular cultural or cohort group. In the case of cognitive–behavioral therapy, or almost any other treatment approach, this might mean taking steps to reduce distractions as much as possible and focus on one idea at a time, proceeding at a slower pace than usual to give the client time to digest the idea fully and make appropriate accommodations, and using various memory aids to solidify the learning, including the use of notes, cards, recordings, and reminder texts, e-mails, or phone calls.

There are clearly other adaptations that therapists must make when working with older clients, regardless of their orientations and preferred models. Kennedy and Tanenbaum (2000) reviewed examples of how practitioners might make such adjustments. Cognitive behavior therapists, for instance, might challenge dysfunctional thinking by understanding older adults' learning styles and memory issues, perhaps including more concrete examples, paper handouts, and written homework assignments that apply the concepts to specific, identifiable, practical problems.

Evan was frustrated with the way his daughter-in-law treated him like a helpless child. He had been living with his son's family after recovering from surgery, but found the experience to be excruciatingly frustrating; he couldn't wait to get back to his own home. The therapist directed Evan to keep a written record of each time he felt upset and then write down notes about what he was aware of, what he was thinking, at the time. Evan quite enjoyed this assignment for the mischievous reason that it felt like he was "tattling" on his family; he even giggled as he went through his list during sessions. The therapist and Evan then spent their time together reviewing alternative ways he might respond internally to each incident. For instance, when Evan's daughter-in-law asked if she could cut up his meat for him, instead of telling himself he was being disrespected, he could instead remind himself that she was only trying to take care of him because of some helplessness she feels in her own life. This helped him to feel more gratitude and compassion than resentment and anger.

A psychodynamic therapist helping an older client deal with survivor guilt and her sadness and grief about outlasting so many of her friends and family members might focus on targeted transference issues related to the feelings the client has toward her younger, relatively "inexperienced" therapist. An interpersonal therapist would operate more concretely with a client, concentrating on specific problem-solving issues rather than the usual underlying patterns that might be more abstract. In a similar vein, any therapist who is used to working at a level of insight would also demonstrate far more patience and flexibility during life reviews and reminiscences to allow older clients to tell their stories without interruption and with much greater patience.

JEFFREY: A CLIENT FROM HELL?

I recall one of the most challenging clients I ever worked with, so much so that I was motivated to write a whole book about "clients from hell" after one particular grueling session. This client, who seemed quite old to me at the time, although she is younger than I am now, would drone on and on and on and on and on and on and on and on and on and on and on . . . and on, without letting me get a single word inserted in her monologue of complaints about how nobody ever listens to her. I would become so bored and annoyed that I would check out as well, barely giving her the courtesy of even pretending to pay attention. She wasn't allowing me to make any brilliant interpretations or deep reflections of her underlying feelings. Heck, she wasn't letting me say anything at all!

At one point I became so frustrated that I actually got up out of my seat, walked over to her, put my hand on her shoulder, bent down so she could look directly in my eyes, and said, "Please stop talking for a minute."

The woman cocked her head, abruptly pausing in the middle of a sentence, and looked startled—and more than a little irritated at my interruption. I had heard this particular story several times previously, so I knew where it was going anyway. In fact, all her stories revolved around the same issue—that her family didn't appreciate her, that nobody seemed to care what she thought, nobody respected her the way she deserved.

If I had a supervisor at the time, I'm sure he or she would have confronted me, pointing out that I was treating her the same way everyone else was in her life. I was not satisfied, nor did I feel I was doing my job, if I wasn't talking half the time. It didn't feel like real therapy to just let her rant the whole session. And I could never get her to end on time—she would ramble on and on and on and on and on and on . . . and on. I'd try everything to pry her out of the chair. I'd stand up and walk out of the room, and she'd still just sit there telling another story. Yes, I figured out so much later that this woman was just so desperate to be able to tell her story and have someone—anyone—listen to her, that this what she wanted and needed most, even if it wasn't what I preferred.

Regardless of the ways we usually like to work in therapy, all kinds of adjustments and adapted strategies are required when working with clients of any unique or specific background. Just as we would use simpler language and more structured techniques with young children, we must also change how we work to meet more fully the needs, preferences, and abilities of clients of any age or culture. We make such a big deal about making our approaches more culturally sensitive and appropriate; this applies equally to the culture of aging clients.

FAMILY SYSTEMS ARE EVEN MORE IMPORTANT

Although we are used to thinking systemically, never is this more critical than working with older clients, and especially quite elderly individuals. We discussed earlier how often it is the family caregivers who are struggling just as much, if not more, than the so-called identified client. This is why one of the first and most important questions for us to ask ourselves is how and with whom do we begin (Fredman & Rapaport, 2010).

Sarah Honn Qualls is a family psychologist who specializes in providing a wide range of mental health services for adults. She is thought of as one of the leading authorities on families late in life, and she created an aging center to prepare therapists to work with older adults. This center provides comprehensive psychological and neuropsychological assessment and treatment services to individuals older than 55, along with their families, focusing in particular on many of the issues that we have discussed related to losses, coping strategies, chronic illnesses, and cognitive changes.

Qualls has been warning about the so-called "silver tsunami" for many years—the increasing number of aging Baby Boomers using more and more healthcare resources when there also seems to be a dearth of healthcare professionals interested in geriatrics. An older person may come to therapy for problems related to depression, but may also have dementia, marriage problems, grief over loss of friends, financial issues, and difficulties with mobility. How many of us ever prepared to deal with so many complex, multidimensional presenting problems? Qualls feels that therapists, regardless of their orientation, need to understand older adults in the context of their living systems.

Often it is the case that an older person doesn't choose to enter therapy, but is coerced to seek help because of issues within the family or frustration on the part of caregivers. In the case of elderly clients with dementia or advanced illnesses, sometimes they aren't even aware that a referral has been made on their behalf. Just as we have been trained to operate systemically with most any client, we initially wonder about the bigger picture in terms of whose behavior is both the cause and effect of others within the context.

Conrad, for example, suffered a right-hemisphere stroke almost 20 years ago and, at age 81, was mostly confined either to a wheelchair or a reclining chair in his home. He lived with this wife, who struggled with her own physical problems, which were magnified by their longstanding marital conflicts that had festered for some time, but became even more dramatic in later life after Conrad became helpless and indigent. He depended on his wife for his most basic needs. She, in turn, sometimes punished him for noncompliance if he did not obey her orders.

If it was only the two of them involved in the situation, it would have been challenging enough, given their degree of mutual hostility and acting out that bordered on elder abuse and neglect. But, there were also many others involved in the situation, including an assortment of both temporary and long-term caregivers and a variety of health professionals. Oh, yes. One more thing: both Conrad and his wife (from a second marriage) both had adult children who had also become triangulated into the their difficulties as a function of their financial dependence. Any decisions made by any one party were ignored or contradicted by others who seemed to have a vested interest in other outcomes. Despite having consulted, or been referred to, a variety of therapists throughout the years, no significant changes took place. In part, this was the case because nobody thought to get all stakeholders and parties together to coordinate a collaborative treatment plan.

Of course this sounds good in theory, but is quite challenging to put into practice in such a way that everyone involved could be recruited to any consensual plan. It takes a particular talent to find ways to extend invitations to family members and others in such a way that they will cooperate.

There are times when it is advantageous to organize "network meetings" with all the stakeholders involved in the client's life (Anderson & Johnson, 2010). Such a gathering can easily devolve into a circus of conflict without adequate control and supervision of the proceedings. Various family members, significant others, and health professionals often have competing interests. Longstanding disputes could be festering for years, if not decades. Blame and guilt can easily dominate the proceedings, with the client caught in the middle.

When he works with elderly clients, Jerry Corey feels a special affinity for them, considering his own advanced age. Although he agrees that the larger family system is critical to any successful treatment, he also finds that group work is an ideal format to work through concerns, regardless of the age diversity in the group.

Corey recalls an older man who attended one of his groups and felt extremely uncomfortable because the other members were so much younger than he was. The man wondered how he could relate to them and how they could possibly understand his experience given the perceived generational gulf between them.

"Rather than allow him to drop out without exploring this concern," Corey said, "I encouraged him to talk to others in the group about how he was different from them and how he did not belong there."

Perhaps not surprisingly, after inviting group members to talk about these issues, the man shifted his perspective dramatically and decided to give the group a chance. He learned a great deal by facing his fears and talking about them—and many others also learned so much from him, finding they all had far more in common than they could have imagined.

"So," Corey concluded from this experience, which has served him well ever since, "the bottom line is that I do not make assumptions, but let older people decide what they want to say about their own lives."

For the reasons that Corey has highlighted, group therapy is often an ideal setting to explore issues related to aging. There is a lot of talk about the importance of cultural diversity in our work and nowhere is this more critical than in creating learning opportunities for people to interact with others representing different ages. Older people have so much to teach younger group members about their experiences; likewise, younger people have much to offer as well.

ASSESSING STRENGTHS AND LIMITATIONS

It is fairly obvious that the evaluation and diagnosis of older clients becomes more significant given their longer life history, likely medical/biological issues, possible impairments or disabilities, and need for consultation with other health professionals and family members. This can also lead to some rather practical things that must be considered to collect and assess functioning accurately. It would be important, for example, to have a complete list of all medications prescribed regularly (or taken). When one of our clients was asked to bring her pill bottles to a session because she was uncertain about the names of all her drugs, she brought a paper bag filled with dozens of drugs that had been prescribed over the years by her various physicians, many of which she was administering to herself in combinations that appealed to her.

It is also important to make sure that elderly clients come to sessions wearing properly adjusted hearing aids, glasses, or other devices that compensate for possible sensory impairments. Appointment times need to be scheduled in such a way to account for any transportation and mobility challenges. And there are issues that may test a therapist's patience and flexibility—when appointments are forgotten or canceled at the last minute.

It helps to call ahead to remind the older client of the appointment. At times, it is necessary to arrange for transportation, meet them at the clinic entrance, and assist them into the building.

One of the first tasks after exploring the presenting complaints with an older client is to evaluate current functioning that may, or may not, be a underlying contributor to the problems. At the most basic level, we want a clearer idea of the person's resources as well as weaknesses. This leads to some rather straightforward questions that we would ask:

- What can you do fairly well?
- What can't you do that you would like to be able to do that is realistic?
- What might you wish to do more often that would make things better for you?
- What would be helpful to stop doing that is wasting your time, energy, and resources?

Marlin was an 86-year-old man who was referred to therapy by his physician because of reported depression. He had a right-hemisphere stroke 30 years earlier and, even after all these years, had not adjusted to his obvious disabilities, which included paralysis of his left side and a host of expected cognitive deficits.

Marlin talked a lot about his desire to go back to work and his interest in buying a company that he might run. Given that he was living on Social Security and didn't know what day of the week it was most of the time, not to mention his limited mobility (he was confined to a wheelchair), this fantasy had become an obsession throughout the latter part of his life. He had been a virtual prisoner of his reclining chair, spending all day watching *Fox News* and old movies, taking naps, and thinking about how he would someday regain the luxurious life he once enjoyed. During the intervening years, he had spent his life savings and retirement income pursuing various miracle cures that might eliminate his afflictions. He had also invested so much of his time, energy, and thoughts planning for a future that was absolutely impossible. Although this provided him with hope and optimism, most recently he was coming to terms with the reality that what he had was all he was ever going to have. No wonder he was depressed.

The therapist spent most of their time together talking honestly about what was now realistic and possible, and what was not. With dwindling finances and, at most, a few years of life left, it was time for Marlin to take stock of his situation in ways he had never done previously. This became the focus of their work together.

When assessments are undertaken and history is taken from someone who has lived a long and full life, a whole new world opens up—a living history of events during the previous century. They have been witnesses, if not participants, in notable historical occurrences—the Great Depression, the Korean or Vietnam wars, Woodstock, and other significant events.

Fred was a vibrant man in his 70s who had a stroke and wanted to train himself to recanalize the blood vessels in his brain and regain his prestroke physical functioning. Fred was hoping his therapist could use hypnosis as a tool that could work with his unconscious mind and allow him to walk better and balance better, and to retrain himself. Along with his wife, he remembered meeting all the interesting people of his era while interviewing them on their daily Chicago radio show. Anyone who was anyone in the world wanted to appear on Fred's show. There was no telling who would stop by when they were in town. Each week Fred would tell his therapist stories about various public figures, whether it was politicians, athletes, Nobel prize winners, scientists, dancers, authors, or stars of stage and screen.

Fred remembered having a cutting-edge scientist on the show who described how the brain was "plastic" and could be healed, or at least changed, with certain interventions. He contacted an eminent psychologist who had appeared on his show and provided Fred with encouragement and some ideas of what he could do in therapy to improve his condition. Although the outcome of the hypnotic procedures produced minimal results—and the therapist still feels remorseful about that—he also feels so grateful for all the amazing stories he heard from Fred during their time together. This experience helped the therapist to appreciate, more than ever, how interesting and fun it was to work with older clients, and it became a new specialty for him. Fred taught him that not only was it important to assess older clients' broad range of strengths and weaknesses, but also do so with himself.

In addition to a life history, more than usual we need to acquire a thorough medical history, as well as have complete access to records. We must ask carefully about sleep patterns, and alcohol and drug use, and of course check cognitive functioning. We also can explore social and family history through family photos, and we are still "old school" in that we find much richer and textural information from actual photo albums brought to sessions rather than digital images on a phone. It is absolutely fascinating to hear the stories and reminiscences that are triggered by sitting on a couch together, leafing through the yellowed pages of photo albums.

Finally, we need some idea of support, resources, and quality of care available, whether from family members or other caregivers. Are the clients' basic needs being met? Are they receiving suitable medical care for their conditions? Are they engaged sufficiently in stimulating activities? Are they in any way subject to neglect or abuse?

EXPLORING COMPLEXITIES

Although there are clear, specialized skills and knowledge required to work with problems in later life, the vast majority of therapists have never taken courses in this area. This is all the more disturbing considering that the issues presented are often far more complex and challenging than those seen in younger clients (Arnold, 2008; Knight & Sayegh, 2010). In addition to whatever presenting complaints are described, there could also be other comorbid illnesses, family issues, pharmacological considerations, cognitive impairments, and sensory deprivations involved. And that doesn't include the cohort-specific knowledge required for that particular generation.

The American Psychological Association (2014) developed guidelines for assessing and treating older adults, in part the result of updating older standards of care, but primarily because most practitioners are relatively unprepared and untrained to work with this population, three-quarters of whom have admitted they need considerably more training. This is especially the case with learning more about polypharmacy and drug interactions, comorbid physical illnesses, cohort generational issues, chronic pain, cognitive impairment, sensory deprivations, and specialized skills for aging clients. And of course, most critically to confront one's own biases, prejudices, ageist attitudes, and personal fears related to one's own mortality and "future self" (Nelson, 2005).

One example of specialized knowledge is related to the values, experiences, and history associated with each of the age cohorts. We may have been required to learn about values of collectivism in Asian cultures, or machismo in Latino cultures, or "tend and befriend" versus "fight or flight" responses programmed by gender, but rarely were we exposed to the unique cultures of each generation. This is all the more surprising considering that, as a function of living so many years and encountering so many experiences, the diversity among older adults is usually much greater than other age groups. Any particular cultural or gender influences can become more pronounced over time, leading therapists to be more cautious about their assumptions. Then there are also the vast differences between different generational cohorts, "the Greatest Generation" of the Second World War versus the Baby Boomers of the 1960s, as one example. Just as we might study the core values and preferences of various cultural groups as part of multicultural sensitivity, so, too, must we become familiar with the unique features and lived experiences that are common to various age cohorts.

In addition, because women live so much longer than men, there are unique challenges faced by older women, who often end up in caretaking roles that have become magnified over time. Aging men, on the other hand, struggle with their own issues related to losing power and control—characteristics that once defined their value.

For those who are members of some minority groups, they may encounter what has been referred to as "double jeopardy." They are more likely to experience economic deprivations and additional forms of oppression because they are members of two disadvantaged groups.

We have covered in various chapters the differential effects of cognitive functioning on an older client's ability to respond to therapy as well as to daily life. There are so many complex and varied issues that must be considered with aging clients that could affect memory, sensory acuity, and cognitive functioning. This can result in psychomotor slowing, reduction in information processing, reduced motor control, and memory retention. And this may be with relatively normal developmental processes. For those with varying degrees of dementia or other diseases, the consequences can be much more dramatic.

Each of these areas that have been mentioned require therapists to have a solid grasp of normal functional ability for clients at various ages and stages of life. This is especially the case with regard to conditions of mental illness or emotional difficulties, especially for those living in long-term care settings. It is not unusual in later life that people might experience once again various psychological problems that visited them in their youth. Depression and anxiety are particularly difficult to diagnose accurately when they are both masked or exacerbated by various drug interactions. In other words, the longer you live, the more complicated matters can become when trying to sort out the sources and causes of problems, as well as their treatment.

PLANNING AND IMPLEMENTING SPECIALIZED TREATMENT STRATEGIES

Although the practice guidelines developed by gerontology and aging experts are intended for clinical settings, they are heavy on recommendations that parallel those for any other group. For instance, therapists are told it's important to interface with other health professionals, behave in an ethical manner, become familiar with the cultural context for their clients' world, apply empirically validated treatments, and so on. They thus serve a useful resource for references on the subject (more than 500 citations!) but offer little practical advice.

At the other end of the spectrum, there are some very specific and precise assessment procedures recommended for elderly clients, adapting mental status exams to this context and population (Hill, 2005). In each case, the questions are adapted to assess cognitive functioning that would be helpful to understand the client's relative abilities:

- What is the date today? (orientation to time and place)
- Tell me what you did yesterday. (memory function)
- What did I ask you a few minutes ago? (short-term memory)
- I'm curious; what do you think is different about you and me? (intellectual reasoning)

- Would you mind writing down a clear statement of what you think your main problem might be? (symbolic processes)
- Would you draw a representation of your family? (spatial reasoning)
- Would you fold the paper into thirds? (gross motor skills)
- What are you no longer able to do? (daily living skills)
- Who helps you do the things you can't do? (social/family resources)
- What are your appetite and sleeping patterns? (self-care)
- Talk about how you feel most of the time. (mood)
- Tell me about feelings of sadness, depression, and being upset. (depression)
- Have you had any thoughts about ending your life? (suicide risk)

Apart from any of these assessment questions, what we are really searching for is an idea about the client's quality of life, regardless of limitations and challenges. Essentially, this means checking to what extent the person is enjoying and making the most of his or her time, and what is getting in the way of improving well-being. Rather than focusing on those things that are not feasible because of physical, environmental, cognitive, or contextual limitations, attention is drawn toward attitude and realistic changes in behavior. Goals can thus be formulated that clarify priorities to concentrate on a few options that are considered most realistic and desirable. As in the case of Marlin, it is also important to abandon goals that are just a complete waste of energy and resources.

Among the therapeutic approaches constructed specifically for elderly clients, Hinrichsen and Clougherty (2006) describe a comprehensive interpersonal model (Weissman, Markowitz, & Klerman, 2000) that has been customized for presenting issues of depression. Consistent with an empirically supported approach, there are fairly specific steps in the suggested protocol, beginning with a thorough assessment during the first three sessions. A series of instruments are administered to check the severity of symptoms and arrive at a working diagnosis. Present and past relationships are reviewed, as well as previous treatments for the disorder. In each case, there is a specific focus on interpersonal functioning and support. This phase ends with a review of medications that may be indicated to manage symptoms.

The next stage, which lasts from one to four months, addresses the identified treatment goals related to four broad areas: grief and loss issues, relationship conflicts and difficulties, role transitions related to aging processes, and skill acquisition. Again, given the relational focus of this approach, particular attention is directed to interpersonal deficits, problems, and obstacles, as well as potential strengths and resources that might be accessed.

The therapist assumes responsibility as an advocate and takes on a far more active, directive role on behalf of the older client. In addition, the therapist might use a variety of techniques to explore salient issues, challenge dysfunctional thinking, facilitate emotional expression, teach more adaptive interpersonal skills, mediate family conflicts, and introduce a number of adjunctive strategies.

In other words, even within the context of this rather specific model, the therapist is far more pragmatic and eclectic than usual.

During the third stage, the focus is on maintaining gains and preventing relapses, solidifying whatever progress has been made, and helping clients generalize results to other facets of their lives. When depression is brought under control there are innumerable opportunities to broaden interests and improve the quality of life in other areas that have previously been neglected or ignored.

LONELINESS AND ISOLATION

It is fairly obvious that just like any unique population, whether based on culture, gender, native language, location, context, presenting complaint, or age range, we must adapt what we do and how we do it to fit the particular needs of older clients. Although we might not ordinarily consider traditional psychoanalytic therapy as the best choice for people in their 80s, a number of researchers and practitioners have been successful adjusting their methods accordingly (Plotkin, 2014; Schachter, Kachele, & Schachter, 2014). For example, Settlage (1996) described working with a woman in her 90s using all the traditional methods of free association, exploration of repressed material, and transference interpretation, and working through intrapsychic conflicts. Obviously this requires a considerable loosening of the traditional analytic stance of remaining aloof and disengaged, because so many older clients long for deep intimacy and authentic connections.

Schachter and his psychoanalytic colleagues recommend a modified therapeutic stance that addresses more specifically issues of isolation and loneliness, as well as more direct and active interventions to help clients reach out to others. The role of the analyst is considerably changed in these circumstances to focus more on support and attachment issues, as well as greater flexibility to work on present-day issues rather than unresolved issues of the past. In addition, after treatment is over, it becomes more important than ever to follow up with clients regarding their actions and outcomes discussed in sessions. Although they speak specifically about the role of the analyst, Schachter et al. (2014) make a compelling point that all therapists have to "enlarge" and expand their roles when working with older clients to deal with their often-persistent feelings of disconnection and isolation.

There are some fairly consistent findings on the value of intimacy, relationships, and social support for older people. Such relational connections can provide an assortment of benefits beyond a mere antidote for boredom or isolation. This includes providing a sense of mastery, empowerment, and personal meaning, as well as a variety of health benefits, such as increased immunity to disease, dementia, and, especially, lower stress levels (Cohen, 2005).

If we do nothing else for our older clients, providing them a space to engage in intimate connection and meaningful conversation on a regular basis can work wonders. Yet, one of the major goals of therapy might also involve helping them to become more actively engaged with the world outside their home and family. This can involve discussions about ways to increase the range of interests and leisure activities, but, more importantly, actually to follow through on these tasks and hold them accountable.

Norton had been extremely active and vibrant throughout his life. After his wife died, he sold his dental practice and felt quite lost. His children urged him to seek some help because they observed him becoming increasingly depressed and isolated. Although Norton reported that the conversations with his therapist were interesting and stimulating, he felt there was really not that much for him to work through. Yes, he was grieving the losses of his lifelong partner and profession, but that struck him as a reasonable response that would just take some more time to process (and he was right). He admitted that he liked the therapist fellow and their time together, but he felt that, because of the therapist's relative youth, he couldn't possibly understand what life was like for him roaming around his home with all the memories of his past. The therapist, however, had made one off-hand observation, followed by a suggestion, that continued to haunt him. The therapist had essentially told him the same thing his children had mentioned—that Norton had to get off his butt, get out of the house, and begin a new life. He couldn't exactly remember how the therapist had gotten through to him, but the one lingering part of their work together was the critical importance of spending most of his days outside of his house, as if that was his job.

It's often interesting how the seemingly most insignificant things we say or do with clients are long remembered far more than the fancy techniques and strategic interventions that are planned so carefully. Norton laughed when he related that, of the dozen or so sessions they'd had together, and all the ways the therapist tried to help him, it was actually one five-minute conversation after their last session was over that stuck with him the most. The therapist had wished him well and then, as an aside, looked meaningfully into his eyes and told him how much Norton had touched him, how concerned he was, and how he hoped Norton would enact some constructive action to take charge of his life once again.

Norton was, at first, annoyed by what he'd heard. He felt the therapist was just meddling, was pushing him just like his own children. Why wouldn't they just leave him alone and let him suffer in peace? But he was later haunted by that last interaction. Or maybe that was just the final shove after all the accumulated input he'd heard throughout their time together, plus the pressure from his family. Regardless, one day, weeks afterward, he work up early resolved to change things in dramatic fashion. First he signed up to join a nearby fitness center and hired a personal trainer to get him started. He started thinking about this as a part-time job and spent a minimum of several hours there each day. Because Norton had some latent social skills, in little time he got to know most of the regulars at the club as well as the staff. After all, as a former dentist he was an expert at talking to people when they couldn't exactly reply when their mouths were full of instruments.

This was just the beginning of Norton's transformation. When he felt in top physical shape, he decided he'd like to see some of the world that he'd missed in his previous life (his wife liked to stay close to home). Although he was perfectly comfortable being on his own, he realized his therapist and children had been right when they urged him to spend more time with others. So, he joined a group of volunteers who were traveling to South Asia, working on a project there to help children. Interestingly, he purposely picked a group of mostly young people because he said he didn't want to be around a bunch of old farts who only talked about their grandchildren.

Norton managed to reinvent himself in later life. Although his therapist will likely never know the real impact he had on his older client, and might even perhaps think the case had only had modest results, it was really the impetus to take action that made the most difference. We mention Norton's case because it highlights how critical it is that we make it a priority of sessions to go far beyond talk and motivate our clients to become more engaged with the outside world, in some cases completely redefining who they are and what they might become.

Cohen (2005) recommends that a therapist's job should be to help older clients develop a "social portfolio" that consists of diversified group and individual activities, especially those that offer a balance between physical mobility and mental challenge, as well as interpersonal interactions. He believes that, just as corporations diversify their holdings to protect against an unpredictable future, so, too, should the aged develop a variety of interests and activities that help immunize them against unforeseen changes. These should include both high- and low-energy activities (community outreach advocacy vs. art projects with children), as well as high- and low-mobility interests (hiking vs. Attending a book club). Likewise, some interests should be structured around groups (theater group or potluck dinner club) and individual pursuits (photography or creating a family history). Cohen believes that such a strategy, if begun early enough, builds assets that can be relied on as a kind of insurance against loss and disability.

MEDIATING FAMILY CONFLICTS

As the therapist packed up for the day, more than ready to head home after a grueling series of sessions without much of a break, the administrative assistant buzzed his office to say there was an emergency and a family was coming in with some kind of crisis. She wasn't sure, but it sounded on the phone as if someone's life was in danger.

Three men, all in their 60s, entered the office a few minutes later and announced quite abruptly, "Our father lost his mind and tried to kill our mother by ripping out her pacemaker."

"Excuse me?" the therapist replied, now paying full attention rather than planning on how quickly he could extricate himself from this sudden situation and go home.

"You heard me," one of the sons answered. "Dad is 94; mom, 83; and a few years ago she had a pacemaker installed. Dad tried physically to rip it out of her chest. We've got her safe now and she's staying with him," and he pointed to one of his brothers.

"Is this a new thing for your parents?" the therapist asked, trying to get his head around what was going on. "I mean, how long have they been married?"

"Actually, almost 70 years. Mom was just 15."

"So this isn't a new thing for them, these kinds of conflicts?"

"Our parents have always been fighting, haven't they?" He looked around and the other brothers nodded in agreement. "They scream at each other a lot—at us, too—but Dad never became physically violent. He's always been, let's say, a rather difficult man for us to love." Again everyone seemed to agree.

Stanley and Iris, the two parents, agreed, with considerable pressure from the family, to visit the therapist. The first thing the therapist noticed was that they seemed quite normal except for the high volume at which they spoke because of mutual hearing problems. The therapist also learned they might have been on their best behavior because a judge had issued a restraining order, forbidding them to go anywhere near one another—an exception was made for this consultation because it was under supervision.

"Let me ask you," the therapist began the interview, "what do you both see is the main problem?"

The couple turned to look at one another, shrugged, and then both tried to answer at the same time, which might not be all that surprising if they'd been together for seven decades. "Our sons are trying to break up our marriage."

"Yes," the therapist replied, disguising his surprise, "they told me things were quite difficult, even dangerous between the two of you.

Stanley nodded his head. "You see, old Iris here," and he pointed to her with a smile, "was trying to drive into town and she can't see a damn thing. Blind as a bat, aren't you honey?"

Iris smiled and nodded.

"So all's I tried to do was pull her arm to get her out of the car, and that thingamajig she's got attached to her chest got disconnected or something.

"Iris?" the therapist prompted, wondering what her version of the story was.

"Stanley's right mostly. I mean, sometimes I can't see too well, especially at night. But I hate asking the boys to do things for me. And I was only going a few blocks to the store. I'm a very safe driver, but Stanley always worries about me." She looked over at her husband as if to say that she appreciated the concern but also found it annoying at times. "I always roll down both widows so I can see better. And I try to listen very carefully before I pull out of the driveway. There's so many cars going back and forth all the time and I sure don't want to hit one."

It was pretty clear that Stanley was, indeed, just trying to prevent an injury, and the whole event seemed to be a misunderstanding that was blown out of proportion. But, that wasn't to say there weren't some major systemic problems in this family.

"I understand the situation better now," the therapist explained, "but your sons also said you fight and argue all the time, and this was just the latest incident that concerned them. When did these fights between you first become an issue?"

They both thought for a moment and then shrugged simultaneously. "I don't know really," Iris said. "Maybe it was during our wedding reception."

Stanley rolled his eyes, sort of saying, "Not that again!"

"Stanley, you see, can be very jealous and he objected with me dancing with other men." She seemed tickled by that.

"Oh, Hon," he answered her, "you know, it's not just that. It's that you looked so beautiful and all them guys were trying to get into your pants. Sometimes you just have no idea."

The therapist spent most of the session trying to keep a straight face because their banter back and forth, rather than striking him as evidence of contempt or anger, seemed to hold so much love and affection. They took turns telling stories about their "fights" together, but they all seemed to revolve around a theme of Stanley being overprotective and Iris trying to get him to back off.

"He can be a pain in the ass at times," Iris said with a giggle, "but he's still the man of my dreams."

At this point the therapist was pretty sure they were not actually a danger to one another. On the contrary, they seemed to have a very loving and supportive relationship. They did argue a lot, it's true, but that seemed to be a normative style of communication for them. When the therapist met with the sons the next day to provide them with a report, they were not at all happy with this assessment and never made contact again.

It was 18 months before the therapist heard from the couple again. Stanley wondered if they could come in for a session with that "younger fella" who, by the way, was himself in his 60s. The couple reported that because their sons were so dissatisfied with what happened before, they insisted their parents see another therapist, who agreed with them that this was a case of domestic violence and that Iris was at risk. Not surprisingly, this led to a divorce and a continuation of the restraining order that they were not allowed to see one another except under professional supervision.

"We're both miserable, Doc," Stanley admitted with tears in his eyes. The therapist looked over at Iris for confirmation and she just smiled sadly and then nodded.

"We miss one another so much," Stanley continued. "We are just living in the spare bedrooms of two of our sons and they treat us like burdensome children. We've tried to tell them they don't understand, that we want to be together, but they don't listen. They think they know what we need, but they never ask us."

"So," Iris interjected, "What my husband is saying is that we wondered if we could schedule sessions with you so we could see one another since this is the only place they will let us meet. Every time I try to tell anyone that we are fine together and that Stanley would never, ever hurt me, that other counselor tells our boys this is just something called 'victim's remorse'; but, if you'll excuse my language, that's a load of poppycock."

"So," the therapist summarized, "let me see if I understand what you are saying. You want to schedule 'dates' with each other in my office because it's the only time your children will let you be together?"

"That's the idea!" Stanley piped in. "They don't like you much, but since we both refuse to go see the crazy guy that they found, you would be our only option.

The therapist (who we now admit was Jon) wasn't sure how he felt about that but, sure enough, for the next 13 weeks Iris and Stanley showed up for their dates. The sons never did agree to relent in their intervention (meddling), and never listened or valued anything else Jon had to say about the case. It was during the third month of their sessions together that they missed their first appointment, which Jon found especially disappointing because he so enjoyed their time together. He later received a message that Stanley got pneumonia very suddenly and died. Ten days later, Iris passed away as well.

It is not exactly unusual that elder family members find themselves smack in the middle of family disputes or part of ongoing dysfunctional dynamics. Children and heirs fight over favored status, if not anticipated inheritances. As we've mentioned previously, caregivers may have their own agendas or problems that compromise their ability—or willingness—to deliver needed services. Whatever ongoing problems had been established earlier in the family life cycle can become more troublesome than ever when an elder member begins to decompensate, potentially destabilizing the whole system. Power hierarchies become misaligned, sometimes thrown into chaos. Historical conflicts, as well as family secrets, can be brought to the surface in unexpected ways. Siblings, children, grandchildren can all become embroiled in disputes during a critical time, giving rise to multigenerational conflicts. Any of these may require the therapist to become involved in mediating these systemic disputes.

The good news is that new models of elder mediation have been developed to address these added responsibilities. Although this also means mastering additional skills, the process begins with a familiar first step of assessing the current structural foundation of the family system, including the communication patterns, power hierarchy, coalitions, boundaries, and intergenerational legacies. Again, it is part of standard operating procedure to engage or join with the family in such a way that we invite each member to share the dominant story that holds his or her perceptions of the salient issues. Narrative family mediation is thus ideal at this stage in that each person is helped to hear and acknowledge the various versions of personal experience. Consistent with this approach, a focus is directed toward strengths and resources within the family unit, rather than identifying only problems and conflicts.

The therapist/mediator's job is not only to acknowledge and value each version of the storyline, but also to conduct a triage related to what requires the most immediate attention. Are safety issues involved? Are there structural realignments that should take priority? How might emotional volatility be reduced? What behaviors within the family should be increased or decreased initially? What has been working most effectively and what has been least effective so far? What entrenched patterns are most likely to prevent new, constructive actions?

Mediation involves a negotiation process during which family members work together toward a common goal, which in this case is better collective functioning to support and help the elder member. This frequently involves learning new skills to resolve ongoing problems, as well as challenging dysfunctional beliefs and myths. As in any other family intervention process, barriers to successful outcomes are addressed, different perceptions are honored, and a consensus is eventually reached that all parties agree to support. Of course the most challenging part of this mediation is not only soliciting promises to support the new way of being with one another, but also actually getting people to follow through on their commitments in a consistent way. This is where things often fall apart, making follow-up and relapse prevention an absolutely critical part of the process.

A SPIRIT OF WONDER

One specialist in geriatric therapy brought his six-year-old son to the nursing home where he worked and the little boy was absolutely fascinated by the older residents, asking questions of them, intrigued by their exotic appearance, and endlessly curious about their lives. Agronin's (2010) son was "bursting with questions," especially after meeting one woman who was 106 years old.

"I beheld the scene of my young son and the elderly woman staring at each other in wonder at the 100 years between them. I saw in my son's face and in this entire demeanor a sense of awe and deep curiosity" (p. 2). And it was precisely this sense of wonder that he considered one of the most "indelible lessons" to guide his therapeutic work in the future. He believes it is curiosity, more than any other attribute and any particular intervention, that helps him deal with the many paradoxes of aging, including the disappointment, fears, and losses, as well as the incredible gifts.

Agronin has come to terms with the challenges of his aging clients by learning to reconcile, if not at least hold, the various paradoxes of their experience. He lists them as a reminder of the wonderful complexity of their lives. Just as they deal with the decline of their bodies, their minds still continue to grow and evolve and mature. As death approaches, they become even more immersed in the present moment. As they cease certain activities and lifelong interests, they also can experience a potential renewal of their lives, learning new ways of finding satisfaction and pleasure. Perhaps most important of all, he has learned that just as aging imposes an "existential vulnerability" on older people that can certainly lead to despair and disintegration, this circumstance can also become the antidote to these exact same conditions. This is also true with respect to the ways that *we* are impacted by our relationship with these clients. There is no doubt that delving into the concerns and issues of older clients requires more than curiosity; it demands a kind courage to face our own most terrifying fears.

Agronin has been surprised by how clueless some therapists are with respect to working with their older clients, often infantilizing, depersonalizing, or patronizing them. It's as if just because we might have a license to practice, and have aged a bit ourselves, that somehow qualifies us to work with this very specialized and somewhat unique population. We have covered earlier some of the myths about aging held by many people, therapists among them, that the elderly are either crippled, dementia-addled crones just hanging around until their death ticket is punched, or else wise sages who hold the elusive secrets of the Universe.

In noting the most common mistakes that therapists make when working with older clients, Agronin first mentions these prejudices and biases that color perceptions and denigrate elderly people, leading to toxic countertransference reactions that would inevitably sabotage treatment with fatalistic and pessimistic prognoses. Second is the confusion often present in complex cases when clients have a long history also affected by interactive social–cultural–biological factors. And third is downright ignorance, which is common when therapists are not intimately familiar with the nuances and hallmarks of age-relevant issues that include retirement, widowhood, losses of friends and relatives, relocations, chronic pain, sleep disruptions, medication effects, and memory problems. He also finds that hubris might be the biggest impediment of all for well-meaning therapists who make assumptions about their clients' experiences based on their own views of aging. This may lead them to see their role solely to facilitate a degree of comfort and adaptation, rather than aiming for ongoing growth and development.

So, here's the bottom line, in case you are still unconvinced: a thorough review of empirical studies examining the effectiveness of therapy for older people concluded that it is indeed helpful in treating anxiety, depression, and subjective well-being, with outcomes quite similar to those for younger clients.

It should be clear that doing therapy with older adults requires specialized strategies and a number of adaptations, just as we would expect with any unique population. At the very least we may have to alter the pace of therapy to take into account slower information processing. This may require other adjustments with respect to voice modulation and tone, as well as physical space. The content of sessions may also be quite different than we are used to, perhaps focusing on a set of different issues related to grief and loss, coping with physical decline and medical conditions, and dealing with challenges of everyday living. We must also function as social workers or case managers at times, looking at presenting complaints within a larger systemic framework of the family. This also brings up a number of unique ethical issues and role conflicts related to informed consent and confidentiality, because family members may have their own agendas and preferences that are not necessarily in the best interests of our older clients.

CHAPTER 12
Death Stalks Us All

When your time comes to die, be not like those whose hearts are filled with fear of death, so that when their time comes they weep and pray for a little more time to live their lives over again in a different way. Sing your death song, and die like a hero going home.

Tecumseh, Shawnee Indian Chief

There is a proverb that has been variously attributed to both Zen Buddhism and West Africa: "When death comes, may it find you alive". Indeed, more than most others, therapists are aware of all the people who shuffle through life as ghosts, barely alive as they are filled with regrets, shame, disappointment, and despair. After all, it isn't death that is so hard, relates actress and writer, Florida Scott-Maxwell (1968, p. 169) "It is waiting for death that wears us down and the distaste for what we may become."

Echoing Tecumseh's quote to head this chapter, and so many other versions of a similar sentiment, there has been a longstanding struggle in every human culture to come to terms with the inevitability of personal extinction. What once seemed far, far in the future becomes a different reality altogether for those in the last chapter of their lives.

SOME VIEWS OF DEATH

Both Sigmund Freud and Carl Jung were dedicated thinkers about the meaning of death and its role in leading to despair or rejuvenation during later life. Although their positions were diametrically in conflict, given their own views on spirituality, they set the stage for many other therapists who followed in their footsteps. Among them, Rollo May (1967) was perhaps among the most articulate early writers on the subject, believing that confronting death in later life was absolutely imperative to promote continued creativity and meaningful productivity. In fact, he believed that death and creativity were closely connected to one another. He saw that, as time became more limited with aging, so, too, did the urgency to come to terms with the greater prospect of life's end.

Victor Frankl, another existential theorist, had his ideas about death forged in the most immersive environment possible—the death camps of Nazi Germany. Frankl (1986) believed that his own constant exposure to death every day, when he watched friends and family members being tortured or starved to death, helped him to come to terms with how precious each moment can be.

James Hillman (1990), a Jungian theorist, wrote extensively on the subject of death, believing that death occurs in a multitude of ways other than one's physical demise. "Each event in my life," he said, "makes its contribution to my death, and I build my death as I go along day by day" (p. 59).

Perhaps most of all, Irvin Yalom has made a career out of exploring the prospect of death as an impetus for living more mindfully. His groundbreaking work on existential issues in therapy (Yalom, 1980) became a foundation for themes he would follow in his writing throughout his life (Yalom, 2006, 2009). Because one of his most significant mentors, as well as his personal therapist, was Rollo May, it is no surprise that he continued his explorations of death anxiety and its meaning along the same lines as his teacher.

In Yalom's (2005) novel about death, he speaks through his protagonist, Julius, who has a terminal illness and less than a year to live, revealing some of his own beliefs about how to manage one's fears. "He would live just the way he had lived the previous year—and the year before that. He loved being a therapist, he loved connecting to others and helping bring something to life in them." It was through his work helping others that his life felt redeemed, just as the prospect of his death became more palatable.

Yalom was especially interested in the ways that, although death eventually destroys us, the *idea* of death is what ultimately saves us. What he meant by that is the prospect of limited time gives the therapist leverage to push clients to take the important, constructive risks they have been avoiding. It is the fear, the terror, of annihilation that gets our attention like nothing else can, hopefully motivating people to take responsibility for their actions and to appreciate better the sacred value of every waking moment.

For older clients (and their therapists), nearing the end of their life encourages far greater urgency to delve into existential issues related to meaning-making; it is one of the major developmental tasks of later life and thus a fertile area for exploration in therapy. In a series of interviews with people in their 80s, those who were most well adjusted and satisfied with their lives tended to be those who had the chance to talk to others about issues related to death (Borglin, Edberg, & Hallberg, 2005).

Let's face it. Death is the most disturbing, saddest, distressing idea imaginable. Regardless of one's spiritual beliefs, or what one imagines happens after breathing ceases, short of reincarnation to a higher life form, death usually means leaving everyone and everything behind, at least in this world, with the next a bit uncertain and mysterious. The only thing that might be conceivably attractive about death is that someday you might be so decrepit, lonely, disabled, cognitively impaired, and in such physical agony, that ending your miserable existence is a welcome relief. For most people, however, they go out kicking and screaming.

In his review of what prominent psychological theorists had written about their views on facing death, Moraglia (2004) concluded that almost all of them have found that "a confrontation with one's mortality is not morbid and inimical to life; on the contrary, it may constitute one of the necessary preconditions for psychological growth" (p. 355). Certainly such explorations will stir up considerable fears and anxiety, but that is not necessarily a bad thing at all if such feelings lead to deeper engagement in life with whatever time is afforded us.

FACING FEARS OF DEATH

Although death represents the ultimate negation of life experience, it also produces some of the most powerful emotional transformations. After turning 62, Susan Sands (2009) felt motivated to explore the ways that death, which knocked more urgently on her door, led to an "expansion of the self" and "pruning of activities." She discovered that all the years she worked as a therapist prepared her to face her mortality better: "The very nature of the work we do helps us negotiate, in a number of ways, the narcissistic crises of older age and impending death" (p. 160).

Sands has noticed all kinds of other ways that aging has provided certain gifts, that she has become far more pragmatic and practical-minded, more guarded in who she chooses to spend the limited time left, more emotionally integrated, and a much better therapist. Despite her "clouded memory" and "falling of the flesh" she has felt validated that there is no better profession in which to grow old. She feels ready to face her death, and help her clients to do so, precisely because she has had so many opportunities to reflect with others on the deeper meanings of life. This is also why she never wants to stop working and has no immediate plans ever to retire.

At age 62, Sands (2009) became quite aware of how different things felt living in her "second home," her therapy office, than during earlier periods of her life. More than anything else, she was accepting that what precious time she had left was taking on a new meaning. "My greater proximity to death brings with it a growing awareness of my own mortality and, if I do not run from it, a greater acceptance of it. As I move inexorably closer to death, it becomes harder to deny its inevitability" (Sands, 2009, p. 158).

She makes the further point that therapists, in particular, are in a privileged position because of the nature of our work to deal with the narcissistic crises of old age and death. Sands believes that, rather than surrendering to fear and despair, we are ideally situated to help ourselves—and our clients—to realize that a greater awareness of the prospect of death can empower us in many ways. We are able to engage more actively and passionately in each moment, and face reality with lowered defenses and an expansion of self. Such potential growth and development can also make us even more successful in our work with others: "Our empathy can deepen and our ability to provide containment can become more effective, encompassing, and reliable" (Sands, 2009, p. 162). This comes from our courage to face what others hide in the shadows.

If death anxiety is not only normal, but expected as we age, then therapists are especially well equipped to help people deal with these fears that can become crippling. Researchers who investigate "terror management theory" call this "morality salience," and talk about the ways people create buffer systems to manage their often-overwhelming unconscious terror of death (Lewis, 2014). There are the standard psychodynamic defense mechanisms that include, most prominently, denial and repression, but may also involve sublimation, displacement, and withdrawal, among others. Then there are other ways that people manage their uncertainty or fears that are more culturally embedded, such as the use of mind-altering substances, workaholism, or belief in an afterlife.

JEFFREY: MY LAST DAY ON EARTH

The Specter of Death has been my companion ever since I can remember. Maybe it all started with seeing so many horror movies as a kid. More likely it has something to do with my mother's cancer and father's heart disease and stroke. When I was in my early 20s, crying at my mother's beside, her attending physician informed me that with my genes I'd be lucky to see 40. From that day onward I have mostly pretended that each day was my last on Earth. Understandably, this has led to a lot of impulsive decisions, impatient behavior, and the determined effort to see and do and experience everything I can, as soon as possible. Any idea that occurs to me, I want to act on right now, just in case I don't get the chance tomorrow. Each night that I go to sleep I consider the very real possibility that I won't wake up tomorrow.

I have had a few close brushes with death, some the result of overzealous adventures (hypothermia, drowning, falling off a cliff, and so on) and others the result of genetic inheritance from my parents (melanoma, heart disease, stroke, lung cancer, and so on). I rarely have felt sorry for myself and, instead, have chosen to think of mortality as a gift that inspires me to live each day as if it was my last. And this belief, this value, has definitely affected the way I do therapy with people of any age.

Death means so many different things to people, depending on their belief systems. I suppose if you believe you are going to heaven, or will be reincarnated in a higher life form, the prospect of ending this existence wouldn't be so disturbing. But if we are honest, everyone has some doubts about whether, ultimately, we will all just be food for worms, whether death represents simply nothingness forever after.

I remember hearing a story about philosopher Bertrand Russell when he was in his 90s, lamenting the ways that most people waste so much of their lives, as if they will live forever. He said he'd like to stand on a busy street corner in London and beg passersby for the precious seconds of their lives they squander and wile away out of boredom or laziness. Ever since then I've imagined that, if Russell had stopped me, I could tell him I had few extra moments to spare.

I think that, more than most, therapists are quite aware of impending death. It isn't just our familiarity with existential themes, but it's also that our lives are so demarcated by small segments of time. Our sessions are usually timed to the minute. So, often, we listen to people utterly wasting their precious time, stalling, hiding, avoiding, denying, making excuses—often really good ones—for why they can't do what they want or get what they want most. We watch the minutes tick by and wonder why some clients choose not to make the most of what they (or others) are paying for.

I think my greatest fear isn't related to dying, but rather to holding on to regrets. I've made some spectacularly stupid and irresponsible decisions in my life that have resulted in financial losses, emotional suffering, and annoyances and additional challenges for my family. And yet I regret none of them. Well, maybe there are a few things I wish I had done a little differently. But, the main imperative of aging that gets better and better is that there is even less time to waste on things that don't really matter. I suppose that is the message I'd most like my older clients to understand.

Those who are able to find, or better yet, *create* meaning in their life are not only better able to deal with their fears of death, but also they are able to achieve a kind of immortality through behavior in later life that leaves a perceived legacy. In addition, developing a sense of meaningful purpose in later years helps people to cope better with life's challenges, reduce the risk of mental illness, manage other health issues, and report a much better quality of life. It is not just that they are in denial about their impending death as much as they are so much better at managing their anxiety about it.

Richman (2006) has been a strong proponent of using humor as a primary means by which to help older clients confront and deal with their fears of death. Woody Allen once famously said that he didn't mind dying very much as long as he didn't have to be there when it happened. He also declared that he had no interest in achieving immortality through his body of work, but rather preferred to do so by not dying at all.

Richman has provided a number of clinical examples of how he uses humor and jokes to help his older clients come to terms with their fears about dying. He cited one case of a 73-year-old man who was terminally ill, severely depressed, and immobilized because he felt there was no time left to accomplish anything meaningful. Richman responded by telling him a story of two friends who greeted one another by asking how things were going.

"Poorly," one man replied. "My uncle is terminal and doesn't have long to live."

When the two friends met a week later, the man was again asked how his uncle was doing.

The man just nodded his head sadly. "The Board of Health refused to bury him."

"Why the hell not?" his friend asked indignantly.

"Well, because he isn't dead."

The client thought that was hilarious. When Richman ended the session by saying, "I'll see you next Thursday, if I live," the client snickered and said in response, "And if not, I'll see you Friday."

Richman explained that this was an example of humor that was introduced spontaneously and customized for the particular situation and context, conditions he considers crucial to make that the intervention both sensitive and appropriately well timed.

It turned out that it was later revealed that the client's fears were not just related to his own death, but also that he would be abandoning his wife, and he feared how she would cope without him. When Yalom (2008) talked about his feelings about the prospect of his own death when this became an increasing possibility, he shared this primary fear that he felt a certain anxiety, if not terror, that he'd be leaving his wife alone.

JON: RETURNING FROM DEATH'S DOOR

I have already died and returned to this world. Since my recovery from almost certain terminal cancer, nothing is different and yet everything is different. I know this is confusing but I'll try to explain. I continue to do all the same things I did before being sick. I teach graduate school, see clients, write, work out daily, play with our dogs, and go to northern Wisconsin during the summer. And yet, everything feels different than it used to. I am not so confident in what I do nor am I sure that what I do is what I ought to be doing. I wonder if I will be alive next week or tomorrow. Is this my last book? What if my mind starts to go or my memory fails significantly? I am starting a new job and people have great expectations that I feel I must live up to. Before, I never considered dying and thought there was plenty of time.

I think of all those who have died before me. I picture their bones in the ground or the ashes spread in the woods. Then I think about what difference does it make, and then to what does make a difference. When I almost died in the hospital a couple of years ago I was at peace with myself and accepted this reality. Now, however, I feel the fear and regret that I ignored earlier. I am trying as hard as I can to practice what I advocate others, to live in the moment, stay in the present, and not allow myself to be pulled into an uncertain future.

TALKING ABOUT DEATH

Contrary to popular belief—or at least practice—it usually helps to talk about feelings about impending death. And that's where we come into the picture as the most logical individuals (besides a member of the clergy) to have that ongoing conversation. Physicians are often quite uncomfortable talking to their patients about the subject because they feel like they have somehow failed when their patients die. This often leaves the families stuck with the job if it is brought up at all. It turns out that it is precisely the invitation to talk about end-of-life issues that is most needed, and therapists are ideally positioned to be the ones to handle those difficult conversations.

JEFFREY: LIVING AND WORKING WITH DEATH EVERY DAY

As I write these words, I am on a plane returning from Nepal, where I spent the past few weeks leading a medical team after the successive earthquakes that rocked the country. During my first day conducting a health clinic, a 7.2 quake literally knocked us down, crumpled buildings, and led people screaming and crying to safety. For the two weeks we were working in remote areas, near the epicenter of the earthquakes in the Everest region, I often slept with my clothes on and a flashlight in my pocket.

I have talked to hundreds of people about death and fear during these past days, not only their terror but my own. Every time the earth shook, we all imagined the end was near. Yesterday, they brought in a three-year-old girl to see me. Her father had just died of a head injury and they wondered how to tell her he was never coming home. They wanted to know if our foundation could provide her with a scholarship because she not only lost her parent, but her home and all their possessions as well.

After they left, I started sobbing in helplessness, still not certain if I was crying for them or for myself. I have seen so much death and despair during these past weeks that I have never felt more alive and yet never more terrified about how randomly any of us could literally vanish into the earth.

We have both talked with many clients about death as they dealt with grieving their losses. We have even worked with those who knew that death was just around the corner for themselves and were busy trying to tie up loose ends and make sure those they love, and those who depend on them, are well cared for.

As we age, we have both noticed how much more seriously our clients actually listen to us when we speak to them about death; they assume we must know something about the subject because we are so close to the end ourselves.

While working in nursing homes, death was a frequent topic of conversation, sometimes in joking ways but at other times a quite serious discussion. What do they think will happen when they die? Who will really miss them? What are some of the things they wish they could stick around to experience or see? Would they consider taking their own lives if the pain becomes unmanageable?

Death was a popular subject to talk about with each of the residents because everyone in the building knew this was their last stop in the journey of life. They realized that death was the next life stage. They readily admitted this was their last home and they would likely never leave the building alive. Some thought the sooner the better whereas others seemed to fight the inevitable ending. A few would visit relatives for a holiday celebration or a weekend and would talk about how much more they appreciated life, which made death easier to accept. As their therapists, we also found these conversations not only enlightening, but also comforting in their own way.

In an article written for doctors, encouraging them to be more proactive in initiating discussions with their aging, terminal patient about important issues, Quill (2000) recommends asking directly a number of important questions that we might also find useful in therapy. We have adapted those we consider most relevant to our work:

- What do you consider most important for you to achieve in the limited time you have left?
- What are some of your greatest fears about what lies ahead?
- Although you are struggling with a number of challenges, what still makes your days worth living to their fullest?
- How could the quality of your life be improved and what steps could you take to make that happen?
- Who have been your greatest models of those you have known, or read about, who had a "good death?"
- If your deterioration continues and you are no longer able to speak for yourself, who would you like to designate to speak on your behalf?
- What instructions have you left as far as a "living will" or your wishes with regard to resuscitating you if and when you stop breathing?
- If you die before you have a chance to complete the things that are most important to you, what would be some of your greatest regrets?
- What can we do to make the time you have left more meaningful and satisfying?

The importance of developing an awareness of death is a fundamental concept of Buddhism. Buddhists believe this awareness offers benefits to the living. It can help release the living from unnecessary attachments that lead to suffering, create compassion for others, put us in touch with unrealized energies, and force us to be more responsible for our actions. In short, an awareness of death can bring about a much greater appreciation for life.

Buddhists believe that death is an absolute certainly that must be acknowledged as early as possible. Life has a set limit and each breath, each heartbeat, takes us closer to that time. The fact is that we are dying from the moment we are born. Our job often involves assisting those who are staring death directly in the face to focus on their own mental and spiritual development.

SOME SPECIAL BURDENS

It is rather obvious that for those who are working with the elderly, we had better get used to facing death on a regular basis, considering the higher mortality rate of our clients. One gerontology specialist, Helen Hudson, disclosed that she had just attended two funerals in the past 36 hours. "Dealing with the elderly," she says, "means preparing for the worst immediately while hoping for the best ultimately" (Irving, 2013, p. 29).

How is it possible to sit and be fully present with people during the last stage of their life, exploring the deeper meaning and purpose of their existence, without doing so for oneself? "I have my own feelings of fear, loneliness, anxiety, despair, and joy," admits Suri (2010, p. 183) in her work with elderly clients, who have helped her to find the courage to look at issues related to her own mortality.

Facing our own fears of death is only one of the burdens when trying to help others deal with their mortality. Scalmati and Kennedy (2009), based on their own extensive work with elderly clients during their last years, identified several other special challenges that begin with becoming drawn into the client's despair and sense of hopelessness. They point out that "it is neither normative nor healthy for anyone to believe that life is not worth living, regardless of age" (p. 835). Our own personal reactions may trigger extreme anxiety, which leads us to buy into this pessimism that is not at all constructive for either party. Of course there is no "cure" involved because death *is* the inevitable end of the journey, but our job is to help older clients focus on the process of their daily existence for whatever precious time they have left. One of the "gifts" of such an approach is that it can very well help us to appreciate our own present moments with greater passion and gratitude. There's nothing like being close to the immediacy of death to help us to live our own life with greater urgency.

Scalmati and Kennedy (2009) also remind us that such intense and emotionally evocative sessions dealing with death issues require even more supervision, teamwork, peer support, and perhaps personal therapy than any other work we might do. If we are honest, it can scare the crap out of us, especially for those of us who are older ourselves.

Most of us remember that awful prayer that children were once introduced to: "Now I lay me down to sleep... If I shall die before I wake...," which, if you pay attention to the actual words, is telling kids that, hey, just in case you die while you are sleeping tonight, you had better prepare your soul for God. That's a pretty terrifying way to put young children to sleep at night. As we age, that prayer becomes an increasing prospect of reality. After age 60 or so we no longer have any right to expect that we will necessarily live another day. This might seem unduly morbid, but many friends of yours may have passed on. More than most, therapists are forced to accept the prospect that we won't necessarily awake tomorrow. This can be a gift in that it has helped us truly to live in the moment and to appreciate better that this may indeed be our last days.

OUR OWN DEATH LESSONS

Robert Wubbolding, who is instrumental in developing and promoting reality therapy, has faced a number of health problems in later life that forced him to look death more squarely in the face. "Having undergone quadruple bypass surgery, treatment for cancer, and other less serious issues, I cannot reasonably expect anyone to fully appreciate what it is like to face the possibility of death. Dealing with serious issues has given me a very different perspective on what is essential and what is incidental."

Wubbolding has found that, recently, he has difficulty managing his time. "My wife and I spend an increasing number of hours attending funerals, visiting people in hospitals, burying relatives and friends, and sitting in doctors' offices waiting for them to attend to our aches and pains." Although not immediately life-threatening, he is frustrated with how much time it takes just trying keep himself tuned up and able to function effectively. One of the "gifts" of approaching death, mentioned earlier, is validated in Wubbolding's experience. "A major lesson that I have learned is to take time to visit friends who are less healthy than I am. Without intending to be morbid, I have learned the visit could well be the last one."

A therapist in his 90s found himself struggling with adjustment to advanced old age, with all its accompanying challenges. He remembered a quote from somewhere attributed to John Dewey that said that every period of life may have its unique difficulties, but also distinct possibilities for worthwhile living, some of them even optimal during old age. Yet he couldn't reconcile the inherent discrepancy between that ideal and the reality that old age is hardly preferable to youth or even middle age. "So Dewey's promise that there are advantages in being old left me doubtful, for he failed to stipulate what these might be, or if he did I had forgotten them" (Leavy, 2011, p. 707).

Trying to be scrupulously honest with himself, and others, Leavy mentions that what is truly unique about old age is that it represents the very end of life. "Anticipating ten years now is extravagant," he confesses, "and I stick to the policy of planning nothing beyond the year ahead" (p. 709). What he has lost, what all of us lose eventually, is the prospect of a future. Consider a life without planning, without thinking about what you will do next year, about what you want to do. We can glorify and romanticize and idealize old age all we want, but the truth for most of us is that it is a time of nostalgia. It is a time of regret. It is a time of grief over all that is lost. It is a time without much time left at all. And as Leavy reminds us, it is a time to realize that we are all what we will ever be.

Leavy isn't trying to be morbid, but he had just lost his wife and life partner and had never felt more alone. He was finally coming to terms with the reality that he had not much of a future left at all.

OLDER PEOPLE DYING YOUNG

Jerry Corey, introduced in several earlier chapters, thinks a lot about how quickly time is passing as he ages and considers that, in just another decade, he will be approaching 90 if he is so fortunate. And Corey is an example of someone who is completely enjoying these sunset years with minimal difficulties. He has a fantasy that he'd like to be featured someday as one of the centenarians who is still active—hiking and biking every day—and still writing books. "It's sobering, though, to realize that I've used up most of my allotted account of years. I do feel anxious when I think about this. I have few, if any, regrets about my life and career, and don't think I have to move any mountains."

As we mentioned earlier, Corey is fairly committed to giving himself the time and space to devote his energy to things that matter the most, being highly selective in ways he would not have done so when he was younger. That's the reality of having limited time left in that we want to make the most of opportunities. One of the ways that Corey deals with fears and anxieties related to limited time and impending death is by staying as mindful and present as he can in his daily life. This is now his greatest challenge because he has been so future-oriented throughout his life. "I would like to get better at fully experiencing the here and now. I realize that I cannot live forever, yet I do think that I can make the most of whatever time I do have. This involves taking the time to reflect on what is most important and making wise choices. I am convinced there is a lot I can do to remain alive and vital, both personally and professionally, even though I advance in age."

This idea by Corey was also a large part of the way that Carl Rogers faced the prospect of death during his later years. Rogers took comfort, not from the prospect of ending up in heaven some day, but rather from the sense of immortality he felt knowing that his ideas would continue to live within his clients, students, and readers. He felt like he would remain alive as long as his life's work would continue to help others. "So I consider death with an openness to experience," Rogers (1980) said, echoing the major theme of his work. "It will be what it will be, and I trust I can accept it as either an end to or a continuation of life" (p. 16).

Rogers had been frail and ill as a child, and doctors had warned him that his life span would likely be short. He was told he would die young. He thought that was kind of amusing because, in one sense, that turned out to be true. Although he lived to a ripe age of 85, he felt he had never grown old and actually died quite *young*!

DYING WELL

Dying is literally the most natural thing in the world. Everything living eventually ends its existence, at least in its present form. This is what permits evolutionary development. You can resist and deny death's inevitability, but it still comes knocking when your time is up.

Dying is easier, or at least less terrifying, when it feels like you have some degree of control over the process. When terminal patients were asked to talk about their own preferences for life's ending, they mentioned most frequently that they preferred to avoid pain, which makes sense that they'd prefer a degree of comfort. Second, they wanted active involvement in any decisions made related to their fate, whether involving medical choices, timing, or conditions. Third, they wanted sufficient time to make their own preparations for the end; this meant finding a balance between sufficient medication to manage pain but not so much that they sacrificed a degree of clarity. Finally, it is not so surprising that it was important they be treated with respect and dignity. If possible, it was also especially appreciated that they were offered some acknowledgment by others of the contributions and impact they made during their lifetime. In summary, the best conditions for dying well included opportunities for closure, feelings (or illusions) of control, interpersonal connections to loved ones and caregivers, preparatory tasks, and a sense of purpose and meaning associated with a life lived well (Munn et al., 2007; Wass & Neimeyer, 1995).

There are some decisions to be made as death approaches, and therapists are in an ideal position to help with these choices involving the identified older client as well as family members (Coppola & Trotman, 2002). Some of these are legal decisions whereas others relate to future medical treatments and financial choices. A number of challenging questions are worth exploring:

- To what extent should life-sustaining medical treatments be used?
- How should living wills, durable powers of attorney, and do-not-resuscitate orders be constructed?
- What treatment preferences and procedures should or should not be considered viable?
- Who should be given surrogate power to make decisions in the event of incapacitation?
- What end-of-life and unfinished business needs to be taken care of?

Although many of these questions may be, and perhaps should be, discussed with legal counsel, they are also valid issues to be explored during therapy. However, one area that would likely not be shared with many others has to do with the ways one would like to go out in preferred style. We are not referring to assisted suicide, but rather to the opportunity to think about a kind of last will and testament that is related to saying goodbye and leaving a legacy for loved ones that is *not* related to money or possessions. This can involve anything from creating a video, audio, letter, journal, document, or portfolio that represents a life's wisdom and experience.

WE INTERRUPT THIS MORBIDITY BY DISCUSSING WAYS TO POSTPONE DEATH

As therapists redefine their roles as lifestyle coaches and proponents of healthy living, we add to our expertise about what most leads to optimal functioning across a broad array of emotional, intellectual, spiritual, and physical dimensions. And it turns out that much of what we might think we might know and understand about what prolongs life may not necessarily be accurate.

Friedman and Martin (2012) spent 20 years following up on Lewis Terman's original study from 1921 about why some people thrive and others wallow in self-pity as they age. More specifically, they were interested in why some people die before their time. They tracked down the original participants in the study, many of whom were now in their 80s, and wanted to know what it was about their habits, attributes, choices, and behaviors that predestined them for long life or one that ended prematurely. Was it related to their genetic inheritance, diet, exercise routine, marital status, colonic enemas, vitamin regimen? Was it something about their personality or even marital status?

After studying the original data, and then investigating the details of the participants' lives, they were first able to identify a few things that were absolutely known to shorten a life span. You could immediately guess what a few of those might be: smoking, substance abuse, and perhaps genetic abnormalities. In addition, they summarized other known factors such as recklessness or impulsivity that would lead to poor decisions and avoidable dangers. In addition, they identified infectious diseases, exposure to combat, radioactivity, ingestion of lead, and, of course, accidents and catastrophes. There is even new research along the horizon that indicates future possibilities of predicting one's life span based on a "DNA clock" that reveals chemical changes over time. It would appear that some people's clocks just run faster than others, regardless of the lifestyle choices they make.

Far more interesting—and revealing—were the predictors of a long life, some of them not necessarily apparent or obvious. First, there were certain personality traits they found associated with long life. Among them, and most prominent, was the characteristic of conscientiousness. This makes sense when you consider that such individuals are far more likely to protect their health, follow doctors' recommendations, avoid unnecessary risks, do things in moderation, and abstain from smoking or drinking. They are the ones who always wear seat belts and develop consistent habits designed to avoid trouble. Conscientious people are also more responsible, dependable, and persistent. They also have healthier relationships and marriages, and enjoy increased success in their careers, bringing additional resources that serve to protect and immunize them against risks that would affect others who are less vigilant.

Long-lifers are selectively and discriminately sociable. They enjoy a solid support system, but one that includes quality, intimate relationships rather than a vast network of superficial connections. They have an optimistic disposition that leads to greater resilience when faced with inevitable disappointments and adversity. Because they tend to believe in what is possible, they engage in more health-promoting behaviors. This also makes them agreeable to be around, as well as inclined to more altruistic behavior.

So far we have largely been talking about internalized, longstanding, entrenched characteristics. But we are in the business of helping people take what they've got and *change* existing patterns to those that are more self-enhancing. It turns out that sociable, agreeable people, those who enjoy greater life satisfaction—and longer lives—engage in some consistent actions that are within reach of almost anyone who has sufficient interest and motivation. Those who watch less television and instead invest more time and energy with friends and family are more content. Likewise, those who demonstrate increased physical energy, whether as part of regular exercise, long walks, or any activity that gets them moving, tend to be happier and live longer. It's also important, according to the Longevity Study, to experiment with new behaviors, take on novel and different challenges, and especially to be involved in some project or activity that helps others. We discuss the importance of altruism and social interest in the next chapter.

The ground that is most fertile for us to work with our older clients centers on one of our specialties: cognitive style. Regardless of whether one follows a theoretical model along the lines of cognitive–behavioral therapy, mindfulness-based therapy, acceptance and commitment therapy, narrative therapy, Adlerian therapy, and dozens of others, each of them has its own unique language for describing dysfunctional thinking patterns, and offers unique strategies for challenging these counterproductive beliefs. Researchers found consistently that those people who are prone to catastrophizing die young. They imagine the worst possible outcomes of many situations they face and then approach them with ambivalence and trepidation. No wonder they are often disappointed.

As we've mentioned previously, and what is easily surmised by practicing therapists, longevity is significantly improved, as much as seven years, by a passionate "will to live" and positive self-perceptions related to aging (Levy et al., 2002). Researchers surveyed people who were middle-aged and, even after controlling for gender, socioeconomic status, functional health, and reported loneliness, found that those who had positive, optimistic attitudes toward growing older lived longer than those who believed that the best of their life was over.

LEAVING A LEGACY

Time takes on a very different meaning as the end draws near. It becomes a more precious commodity. This realization is a gift of sorts in that, each day, each moment, can take on a new and different meaning. Time has particular meaning for a surgeon, because a patient's life very much depends on the doctor's swift work opening and closing a wound before infection sets in, or anesthesia-induced unconsciousness becomes potentially life-threatening. In writing about his concept of time, Paul Kalanithi (2015) noted that his work as a neurosurgeon was all about measuring time, which takes on a surreal quality in the operating theater because the moments seem to disappear as a result of the intense focus required. Yet, when diagnosed with terminal cancer at age 36, and realizing he would never see his infant daughter grow up, nor would she ever remember her father, he understood that time took on a very different dimension. The prospect of impending death slowed him down considerably. Although he once raced through his days, like an oldster he now considered himself a tortoise rather than a hare: "I plod, I ponder, some days I simply persist."

Kalanithi wanted to leave something behind for his infant daughter, something she might remember about him. He wanted to leave her a message, so he created his last words and testament, his most important life lesson to leave behind. And this is it: "When you come to one of the many moments in life when you must give an account of yourself, provide a ledger of what you have been, and done, and meant to the world. Do not, I pray, discount that you filled a dying man's days with a sated joy, a joy unknown to me in all my prior years, a joy that does not hunger for more and more, but rests, satisfied." Kalanithi died soon thereafter he wrote those words to his daughter, his most importantly legacy.

Of course we are all dying. And our days are numbered, our moments finite. And all of us, at least those who practice therapy, wish to leave behind something meaningful and poignant, something that makes a mark, something that means something to the world and the loved ones we leave behind.

CHAPTER 13
Dreams Lost and Dreams Found

Beautiful young people are accidents of nature, but beautiful old people are works of art.
Eleanor Roosevelt

What does it mean to have a life that is well-lived?

First of all, it would feature feelings of productivity and the fulfillment of significant goals, of having made some kind of difference. It would mean receiving acknowledgment and recognition of these contributions, with accompanying good memories of the past. Finally, it would involve having enjoyed meaningful relationships.

We also asked prominent therapists what it means to practice exceptional therapy, another variant of a well-lived life related to professional success and satisfaction (Kottler & Carlson, 2008). As you might imagine, there was a wide range of answers reflecting their different backgrounds, values, priorities, conceptual models, and specialties. Some practitioners defined their finest and most satisfying work represented by cases that confirmed their favored theories. Some therapists liked their work most when outcomes were fast and efficient whereas others much preferred long-term relationships with deep intimacy.

In many instances, there was congruence between what they considered a good life for their clients and similar goals for themselves. Those who stressed clear and logical thinking as the secret to a well-lived life tried hard to practice those strategies in their own daily existence. Likewise, those who affiliated with feminist ideals, or psychodynamic principles, or any other therapeutic approach, often committed themselves to apply these concepts to enhance the quality of their own life. We found this both inspiring and validating, considering that practicing what we preach to others is the hallmark of a true master therapist (Kottler & Carlson, 2015).

ON REGRETS

It is pretty easy for any of us to look back on all the things we wish we had done differently, the alternative paths we could have taken or decisions we could have made, the impulsive things we've said and done that we can't forget or forgive. For those who are older, it is sometimes even more difficult to let the past go, especially if it feels like that's all that is left. It is strange indeed for someone to find him or herself only having something interesting to say when it refers to events that happened so many years ago. More and more often, we find ourselves telling stories about work we've done, or experiences we had, decades ago, although we still maintain pretty active and exciting daily lives. With a focus on the past, we remember the triumphs and joys, but also think a lot about the mistakes and failures. So it is the same with our older clients.

It has been suggested that regrets have no adaptive value, but we disagree. As long as you remain stuck in the past, you don't have to deal with issues in the present and future, especially when they feel much less enticing than prior experiences. Regrets often provide opportunities for learning and growth. In fact, studies of the brain show that the orbitofrontal cortex is tasked with the function of comparing imagined results with actual outcomes, which can actually be quite helpful as a reasoning process. That's why, among all the negative emotions that are experienced—guilt, worry, anger, fear, and shame among them—regret is the one that is actually most prized (Saffrey, Sommerville, & Roese, 2008). Researchers have found that people most appreciate how regret helps them make sense of past experiences and gain a deeper understanding of their motives, needs, and desires; and can lead to greater social harmony. Thus, regretting lost dreams and opportunities does not necessarily mean that poor decisions were made, because timing, readiness, and context all matter as well. Sometimes owning regrets help us to make more informed decisions in the future.

Roese (2005) found that people are most inclined to regret opportunities they passed up for further education or career advancement, followed by mistakes they made in romantic relationships or parenting responsibilities. Furthermore, this doesn't change much in later life as these lost dreams continue to fester. The therapeutic goal, then, is to help older adults to let go of past regrets and instead to create new narratives that focus on turning points that led to constructive action based on prior mistakes (Kray et al., 2010).

One therapist who does workshops on the subject of regret has found that 80% of his participants admit to regrets about lost dreams, especially among older people (Kashdan, 2008). He contrasts this with studies of young children who have not yet developed this capacity and let go of things that don't work out the way they wished. He quotes the lyrics of a punk rock band from the 1980s with the distinctive name The Butthole Surfers: "It's better to regret something you've done, than to regret something you haven't done." This is consistent with the research he has studied that regrets linger much longer for things left undone and unsaid than mistakes of the past.

Regrets provide us with leverage when working with older clients. Although they may attempt to minimize or disown lost dreams and regretful behavior, we can use such unrealized desires to deal with unfinished business and motivate action: "It is not too late, after all, for you to take care of some things that are still really important to you."

Of course there are differences between regrets over things you have done versus opportunities that were passed up. It's usually far more difficult to change things that have already happened, and rectify them, rather than following through on dreams that are not actually lost, but merely avoided or postponed. This is one of the most useful and significant tasks that we accomplish in therapy, with young or old, helping them to discover meaning and useful lessons in their regrets and failures.

FINDING OR CREATING MEANING

When it feels like all you have left are your memories, it is easy to become self-absorbed and full of self-pity. Yet many older people find meaning and purpose in later life by finding a cause or project that continues to inspire them. They devote their time helping friends or neighbors, or they engage in volunteer work. One client in his 80s, Morris, drove his wife crazy because he was bored and sat around the house all day. She sent him to therapy to work things out. During his sessions, he was persuaded that he was not too old to pursue his dream of working in a hospital. Although he once imagined himself in the role as a surgeon, he instead found volunteer work as a greeter on the intensive care ward of his local hospital, quite content to support family members of patients who were in recovery.

It would seem that much of the depression experienced in old age has less to do with physical decline and more to do with lacking purpose. As people age, they often have more leisure or discretionary time and do not know what to do with it. We have seen how their self-esteem suffers because they feel invisible and slighted. In the influential McArthur Foundation Study of Successful Aging, researchers discovered that more than three-quarters of older people believed that life wasn't worth living if you weren't actively engaged in contributing to the well-being of others (Gardyn, 2002). This conclusion has also been supported by studies that look at the effects of altruism, volunteering, and prosocial behavior in later life, finding that those who are actively engaged in helping others in some form of meaningful engagement are far more satisfied with their lives.

"The fear of growing old and the fear of death will not terrify the person who is certain of his immortality in the form of his children and in the consciousness of his contribution to the ever-growing culture." This observation by Alfred Adler during his own last years helped drive him to discover the value and importance of his concept of "social interest." He believed that as people grow older, they need time to expand their interests. He noted that "just the reverse happens in our society; we give old people no opportunity for self-expression . . . . This is a pity because they could accomplish much more and would be infinitely happier if they had more of an opportunity for working and striving" (as cited in Ansbacher & Ansbacher, 1962, p. 445)

Adler was vehemently opposed to putting old people "on the shelf" during a time when they still had so much to offer. As such, he didn't believe in the idea of "retirement," but rather that older people should make different choices about how they remain productive. He was among the first in our field to talk specifically and passionately about the importance of social interest, which he called *gemeinschaftsgefuhl*—meaning, "community feeling" in his native German. He equated such an altruistic drive with feelings of self-worth, especially as he reached his later years and appreciated how important it was to give back to others with a sense of selflessness. Foreshadowing Erik Erikson's last stage of life, Integrity versus Despair, Adler believed that healthy adjustment to later life was directly related to feeling a deep sense of purpose mentoring and helping others, whether in the context of volunteering, grandparenting, or devoting one's time to a social or political cause.

In later life, Adler was consumed with getting his message out to the world. He had served as a physician during the First World War, and he observed firsthand the horrors of violence in the trenches. He believed his ideas were necessary if people were going to coexist in peace, and create and maintain balance in life without the need for conflict.

Similar to the other grandparents of psychotherapy at the time, including Sigmund Freud and Carl Jung, Adler would begin most of his days in later life with writing tasks, followed by seeing patients and spending time with friends. He would then hold court in one of the many Viennese coffee shops. The tables would be pushed together and all were welcome to join. Jokes and stories were shared as well as deep discussions about topics such as the meaning or purpose of life. Many would come specifically to listen to him discuss his theory of individual psychology, with its emphasis on social interest.

Even Adler's vacations were actually periods of concentrated work for him. He was an astute observer of himself, as well as others, eventually realizing he was on a self-destructive path. Unfortunately, death claimed him before he could take more constructive action to slow down the pace of his life. To the very end, Adler lived his life with great meaning and purpose. He tried to educate the world about the importance of helping others, although he seemed to have forgotten to help himself.

Adler was deeply distressed in his later years. He had lost many of his closest friends and colleagues during the Nazi invasion of his country. When he learned that his daughter and her husband had died in a Russian *gulag* after years of imprisonment, he became inconsolable. Nevertheless, he managed to conceal his worries and grief by feverish activity.

During the last years of his life, Adler had begun to ponder anew the meaning of life. He gave faith and metaphysics far more weight than he would have been able to ten years earlier. More and more, his ideas circled around the creative powers of man—of every person and not just the artist. He concluded that the development of social interest was the solution for the world's crises. "Who can say where these partly new and unfamiliar thoughts would have led him? Who can say whether this sixty-seven–year-old man would have invited a new breakthrough—that breakthrough with which a human being gives his life an extra dimension that most people yearn for in vain, without which our fragmentary life often degenerates into a wretched piece of rubble" (Sperber, 1974, p. 126).

Before his death at age 67, during the last month of his life, he delivered 56 lectures in four different countries. Obstacles did not exist for him; Adler principle was that they occurred only to be overcome. He grew stronger with growing difficulties or, as it is said today, "What doesn't kill you makes you stronger." However, for Adler, this was no longer the case. Adler was an undersize second child who tried harder to outdo the firstborn child. His compensation and struggle to achieve cost him a longer life. He died of a massive heart attack while out for a walk, but at least he died on his feet, pursuing the passions that defined his work and life.

WHEN IT'S TIME TO QUIT

Although much of our discussion is related to how therapists can rise to the occasion as they age, exploring novel and different ways to use their experience and wisdom, there is also a time to let some things go and accept the limitations that age presents. Sigmund Freud, for instance, did not exactly age gracefully. As his cancer and physical maladies began to mount, and his country was torn apart by the Nazis, he felt adrift. If possible, he became even more pessimistic, critical, and cynical about the future, obsessed with his own losses and declining health (Thompson, 1991). We can't imagine he was a whole lot of fun to be around during these last years.

There is a point for all of us when we may lose the clarity and objectivity to assess whether we ought to continue accepting responsibility for others' care, given the challenges we might face with the multitude of physical compromises we make as we age. This is coupled with other losses as well, including spouses, partners, lifelong friends, status, and power. Some professional organizations, such as the New York Psychoanalytic Society, urged members older than 65 not to accept new patients, a policy that Fieldsteel (2011) agrees should be at least given serious consideration. Full retirement may certainly not be for everyone, but she gave careful thought to the ways her own abilities had changed over the years. There is little doubt that there would be tremendous loss associated with giving up what has defined our identities for so many years, but Fieldsteel doesn't see it as surrendering her profession as much as choosing to apply those skills and knowledge to herself, rather than only serving others. After all, there is plenty of work to do in this stage, with coming to terms with the meaning of our life's work: "We have a rare opportunity to redefine ourselves and our history from a unique perspective" (p. 14). Fieldsteel accepts that she is far more than her role and identity as a therapist. Although she will never stop *being* a therapist, that is not necessarily related to seeing clients actively. She will always continue thinking, analyzing, problem solving, processing, and relating as a therapist because those abilities and experiences have become embedded in her soul.

Obviously, memory is the key resource of a therapist, and when that starts to go, we lose our ability to retrieve relevant information, hold on to key material, make significant connections, and access resources. The speed of cognitive processing begins to decrease noticeably by age 40 and is cut by 50% at the age of 70. This means not only slower reaction times, but also more frequent errors, reduced sensory input, and compromised cognitive functioning (Fonagy, 2009).

JON: I'M NOT AS GOOD AS I USED TO BE

To be honest, I am not as interested in my clients as I once was. I once thought that I would work with my clients throughout their entire lives. As a family-oriented therapist, I saw my role as helping people to navigate the life challenges they would face at various stages over time. Now that my days are numbered, I know I will not be around for their lifelong guidance. I also notice that I am making more and more mistakes related to remembering details about my clients and their problems. I have memory lapses and forget what I want to say, or why I thought something was important. I sometimes say things I think are quite clever, but they seem to make little sense to my clients. I forget what I asked them to work on between sessions and then write it off by thinking it's just because I'm tired—but fatigue is now a constant companion.

Today I looked into the waiting room full of people and couldn't figure out which one was my client, although I knew this was our third session. I was able to recover after a few moments of hesitation, but this is just a reminder of what I've lost.

I've cut down my practice from six days a week to only two, and soon I plan to cut back further to just a handful of clients. I know the end of my work as a therapist is soon coming to a close, and I mourn that as one more loss, one additional surrender of my professional identity. My clients and students tell me I am important to them and they hope that I do not plan to retire anytime soon. I joke that maybe when I'm only functioning partially as an experienced therapist, I might be better than a fully functioning novice. Some days I'm not so sure.

Older, somewhat impaired therapists, or at least those not operating at optimal levels, are allowed to continue practicing because people make excuses for their lapses based on their venerable status. They may drift off or even fall asleep during sessions, become forgetful of important details, and confuse clients with one another. Often, older therapists may not stay current on the latest research, technology, and advancements in the field. In fact, we have heard many older colleagues boast about their refusal to learn new innovations, preferring to stick with what is familiar. This begs the question: How do you know when it's time to quit?

Some older therapists may realize that it's time to quit, but economic realities or a lack of other interests leads them to remain active way past their "shelf life." Sometimes it is quite evident they have lost their passion and interest; they no longer remain current in the latest research and standards of practice. Because therapy is such a private and secluded activity, it is often difficult to know just how effective other professionals may be. And it is sometimes problematic to rely solely on what their clients report was most helpful.

We each have an ethical responsibility to "own" our age and understand the accompanying changes and their consequences. There is a reluctance in our profession, as there is in many others, to confront colleagues about their less than stellar levels of competence. Although we are ethically mandated to do so, the reality is that many may feel it is none of their business, as long as nobody is being hurt (too badly). Liebenberg (2011) became increasingly aware of fellow therapists whose advanced age was clearly compromising the continued effectiveness of their work. She observed that one guy had been running the same group for 20 years with no change in membership during that time, leading her to wonder how much therapy was really going on. Another therapist she knew was treated as a kindly old man who was indulged rather than actually listened to. After he had a heart attack, he started seeing his clients at home to make it easier for himself, but that convenience only eroded his professionalism even further.

Liebenberg mentioned other elderly therapists as well, those who were hard of hearing, who had memory lapses, chronic pain, fatigue, and other problems, all of which they seemed in denial about because of narcissistic needs. Still, she suggests that ending a practice is not necessarily grim; it can be a kind of celebration and honoring of those we have helped, and the clients from whom we have learned so much.

LEARNING TO LET GO

Like many other aspects of life, David Seaburn had to *learn* the skills of retirement and ending his practice as a therapist. Now that he was no longer controlled by his day planner, with every hour of his life partitioned into scheduled

JEFFREY: DID I MENTION MY MEMORY PROBLEMS?

Aging is the issue of our lives, with all the accompanying challenges. For me, it is a lot about memory loss, about no longer being/feeling attractive, about compromises in what I do, about sleep loss, about uncertainty related to the future, about an absence of ambition, about confusion connected to what I want to do with the time I have left, about acceptance of lost dreams, about helping as many people as I can, about coming to terms with dying slowly, about my mortality. Did I mention memory loss?

There are startling reminders of my body's decline and deterioration. My vision is changing, requiring reading glasses. Every time I take a shower I see the remnants of hair falling out, collecting in the drain, far more than will ever be replaced. Limited bladder capacity compromises my sleep. But worst of all, for a therapist, are the memory issues. In my youth I had the most remarkable visual memory. I could see a film or read a novel and practically review the whole story, scene by scene; now I have a 10-year rule: any movie I haven't seen in 10 years is just like watching it for the first time. I used to be able to recollect the smallest details about my clients—the names of all their children, their pets, and whatever they talked about during the previous handful of sessions. Now I must write everything down, which is also a problem because I can't read my handwriting. I repeat myself in sessions or the classroom and I catch those looks that tell me I told that story before. In fact, now, one of my most recurrent questions is: "Have I told you this before?"

It startles me to look in the mirror and sometimes see the mask come down. I look like my grandfather! How the hell did that happen?

I find it increasingly challenging to keep up with all the technological changes and all the energy invested to stay current with the latest innovations. I find myself complaining about how things aren't like the good old days when everything seemed simpler. Oh! And did I mention my memory problems?

sessions, he was overwhelmed with questions that were not dissimilar to what he'd been asking his clients all these years: What would he do next? How would he spend the time he had left? He wondered whether he would "end up forever on the platform watching the train whiz by, its cars full of eager, driven, productive people who are still utilizing their talents and reaching their goals" (Seaburn, 2013, p. 80).

Eventually, he learned some things he'd never mastered earlier in life: how to wait, how to listen and watch more carefully. This was hardly an easy assignment for someone whose life had been so busy and packed most of the time. He spent the first year after retirement confused and anxious, uncertain about the future, until finally a vision began to take shape of who and what he still might become. In part, his toddler granddaughter helped him achieve some clarity when he began to reenvision the meaning of time. When he had been her age, he didn't know that such a thing as "time" even existed. Then, in his teenage years, "time [stretched] out before me like an endless red carpet I could walk down forever" (Seaburn, 2013, p. 79). Finally, he began to realize in old age that time is something far more fragile and delicate, something that, more than ever, must be cherished in such a way that he feels more grateful than ever for every "molecule of experience."

Seaburn's experience is echoed by another therapist who was approaching the end of his life. Samuel Atkin (Atkin & Atkin, 1992) kept a journal during the last years of his practice, when he was well into his 80s, reflecting on what it meant for him to be old. Approaching 90, he admitted that everything was slower for him. He needed a walker to get around. His eyesight, his hearing, even his voice, the instrument of healing, had lost much of their power. His journal read like a horror show, documenting his insomnia, bowel difficulties, Parkinson's symptoms, anemia, and a bunch of other conditions we've never heard of before. Then there was the helplessness and despair he felt. "A weak old man dies ten thousand deaths," he wrote. "He dies every day as his vitality ebbs away" (p. 4).

One of the incredible benefits of spending a life helping others to deal with their challenges is that therapists are well equipped to confront their own infirmities—if they have the courage and resilience to do so. Atkin did not want to surrender to his depression and misery, nor did he wish to continue feeling sorry for himself. Approaching his 90th birthday, he came to terms with his place in life—and the prospect of impending death—accepting what he couldn't change and adopting a new attitude. He realized that, just because the culture of youth likes everything so fast, didn't mean that going slow was a loss, or even a weakness. He rediscovered his sense of wonder at new discoveries, new awareness of unique and different experiences. "Not only is my past relived more vividly and more often than before, but, as already described, my present is lived more intently" (Atkin & Atkin, 1992, p. 14).

These are the enduring residual gifts from our clients. We spend a lifetime in conversation with people about the most thorny, disturbing issues that anyone could ever confront. We lived a thousand lives through the stories we heard—and shaped—in our offices. We had access to the innermost experiences, struggles, and secrets of clients during the most critical transitions of their lives. We accumulated a storehouse of memories that were stockpiled from all that we learned, the mistakes that people made, the failures they faced, the gifts that they offered us through their trust.

A COUNTERPOINT ABOUT NEVER LETTING GO

Age, itself, is a moving target, redefined in light of biological and cultural evolution. Reaching the ripe age of 25 was quite an accomplishment during Stone Age days. Just a century ago, 50 was considered elderly. Yet, adolescence is now extended beyond biological puberty. People now take longer to complete their education, postpone marriage well into their 30s or longer, and change careers multiple times during their life span. Laura Carstensen (2011), one of the premier scholars on longevity, believes that humans catch a "second wind" once they hit 50 "in which the first fifty years of life could be spent learning and shaping ourselves into the kind of people who can spend our next fifty years giving back to our communities" (p. 70). She believes this is a radical departure from the previous script, in which it was assumed the only thing that awaits us at the fifth-decade milestone is a downward spiral toward irrelevance and invisibility. Things have now changed such that some people don't really hit their stride until later life.

Phil Kirk, a 68-year-old therapist, wondered if the traditional model of retirement is even appropriate for what we do, considering that we continue to feel so much responsibility, if not obligation, to continue helping others and giving back to the community. And yet, with more discretionary time, Phil was able to be more focused and selective in the ways he is most helpful. He continuously asks himself: "Am I most effectively capitalizing upon my life experiences and using my acquired wealth of knowledge to be most beneficial to those with whom I work? Should I reevaluate the benefit of self-disclosure and sharing more of my life in helping others? This perhaps sounds somewhat arrogant, but clients respect wisdom and lived experiences, and want to know their therapist is real."

Rather than feeling stuck at this stage of his career and life, Phil sees this stage as "an exciting opportunity not only to use life experiences, but also to enjoy the inherent sense of helping others through finding ways to tap into the wisdom and strengths that life experiences provide." This has given him more self-acceptance and greater confidence in what he does and how he does it. And it has been his experience that clients, and other people in his life, feel inspired by the passion and excitement he continues to demonstrate in his life—and model for others.

AND NOW WE BECOME VERY PERSONAL

We depart from our usual narrative voice and prose to share some personal reflections on what we learned during the past few years that we have been investigating therapy over 50 and working on this project. We intend to be as honest and open and forthright as we can, disclosing some of our own insights and revelations that we hope to pass on as elders within the profession.

Jeffrey: Reconceptualization of What It Means to be Old

I (Jeffrey) acknowledge that this could be reconstructed memory, but I swear (to the best of my recollection) that I recall once reading an article 25 years ago and thinking to myself how disconnected I felt from the subject. For many years I used to read my favorite journal, *Psychotherapy*, from cover to cover. This was rare for me because I've found many other publications may provide only a few pieces of direct interest to me. When I was researching articles for this book I came across a study (Zivian et al., 1992) that reported therapist attitudes toward treating elderly patients and I remember (or believe it so) briefly skimming through the pages after seeing the title that had little interest and relevance to my life and work. After all, I was in my late 30s and couldn't imagine I would ever be elderly, much less have the slightest interest in the issues that concern this population. And now I'm here! And I now wonder, almost every day, where my life went! How did I ever get so old? And so quickly?

Jon: "Just What I Need, Another F*%@#g Growth Experience"

I've already talked about my diagnosis of terminal cancer when the doctors gave me less than a year to live. There was a cascade of other medical issues that followed—multiple infections, a quadruple heart bypass, stem cell transplant, other major surgeries, and the ever-present chemotherapy that led to other systems in my body falling apart. I was literally a zombie, a shuffling shell of what I had once been, having aged two decades in a year. And yet because I never gave up on myself, my oncologist never gave up on me either. I would make the most of whatever time I had left. I would spend quality time with my family. I would complete the latest book project that Jeffrey and I were working on what would become my swan song, my last testament containing all the wisdom I wanted to leave behind about what makes a therapist extraordinary.

Thanks to the miracles of medical science, a lot of luck, faith, and determination, I proved the odds wrong and survived the cancer (so far!). Now, as I begin my 71st year, I think of little else. I worry how much longer I will be able to keep up with the pace of my life. I have less and less energy to do the things I love the most.

After being forcibly retired from my university professorship, I decided to find another job (Jeffrey thinks I'm crazy). I do wonder if I can really manage my new and increased responsibilities, especially when I feel a certain doubt that is only reinforced by so many others who are constantly asking me if I'm really okay.

There seems to come a time when people no longer expect you to be alive and well. Hearing this day after day becomes another challenge, and I imagine it will only get worse the more I'm treated like a relic. Even when I try to counteract others' concerns, I wonder what it is that they see in me. Is it my walk? Are my clothes on correctly? Are there food stains on the front of my shirt? Just what is leading them to think this about me? It is the beginning of a paranoia that is leading me to think and feel that maybe I no longer belong here in this life, that my time to be productive has expired and I need to step aside.

I am learning to recognize that there are times I need to ask for help. I also realize there are just some things I can't do anymore. I'd like to say that I accept these losses, but, truthfully, I've been fighting against them, and myself, every awkward step of the way.

Although it is true that I am slower at getting things accomplished, and I do make more mistakes and forget things, I also seem to have more compassion and deeper empathy for my clients than ever before. I notice that I am able to sift through a lot of information and find what is really important; I notice patterns of behavior and seem to provide deep insight or wisdom when needed. I find I am more tolerant and accepting of some things I used to fight previously.

Jeffrey: "I Don't Have to Do This"

I'd always thought that aging was a relatively gradual, incremental process that proceeded in an orderly fashion from one stage to the next. I've taught courses in human development throughout the years so I'm more than a little familiar with all the theories and research on the subject. So I was quite dumbfounded to discover that, in a ridiculously short period of time, I became old. I turned 65 this year and it seems like, more than any other birthday, this is the one that really got my attention. My body is indeed slowing down and my mind is not what it used to be.

Like Jon, I have come to accept that there are some things I can't do any more. I just don't have the energy or the motivation to work that hard anymore. I feel much more selective and discriminating about how I want to spend my time. I feel the clock ticking down and realize that if there are still some things I want to do, I had better get going. I don't take for granted that I will necessarily be around all that much longer. I noticed that, while doing relief work in Nepal after the successive earthquakes, I simply accepted that the earth might swallow me up at any time, or that I might contract cholera or typhus from all the decay of dead bodies. I accepted this reality almost without complaint or that much concern—okay, maybe a little concern.

I've had more than my fair share of adventures in my lifetime, living in a half dozen different countries and climbing mountains around the globe. I've even done a little bit of technical climbing on Mt. Rainier and some trekking peaks in the Himalayas, but I figured if I wanted to summit a really big, challenging mountain I'd better do it quick. So, I took it upon myself to prepare for climbing some 19,000-foot volcanoes in Ecuador.

I started training for the expedition with ferocious commitment, increasing my workout regimens several hours each day. I "invested" in mountaineering equipment so I'd become comfortable with my boots, crampons, and other stuff. I spent hours on a stair climber with a backpack full of books on my back. I planned my acclimatization to high altitude with careful and meticulous incremental adjustments. After all, I'm not a young man anymore and I wanted to survive this experience more than I needed to summit the volcanoes.

Things did not quite go according to my plan, in that my guide turned out to be more interested in getting me to the top than being worried about my safety. For some reason, he felt competitive with me, and seemed to take pleasure out of shaming and cajoling me to go faster and harder. We began the summit of Cotopaxi at 9 p.m. from base camp, having to start several hours earlier than usual because of closed facilities at the preferred staging point. As we climbed up, up, up, I tried to get in a rhythm that felt comfortable, a task that was became increasingly challenging as we ascended higher, and I felt my guide pulling me on the rope, teasing me into going faster. It was dark—our trail was lit by headlamps directed only at the next few steps ahead—but when I looked off to the side, I could see we were scaling a narrow ridge that dropped off thousands of feet into an abyss. (Did I mention I'm afraid of heights?)

My breathing was becoming ragged and I felt light-headed as we topped more than 18,000 feet. It had started snowing and we lost the trail, so we just headed up the ridge. Hours and hours went by and I trudged on, asking myself why, exactly, I was doing this. It was about 3 a.m. when the voice in my head became more strident, a whisper turned into a scream: *You know, you don't have to do this!* It felt like I was hallucinating. I could barely catch my breath. My legs were still shuffling along, my ice axe clenched so hard in my hand that it felt like a part of me. I kept rehearsing how I would arrest my fall when I slipped off the glacier, a very real possibility considering how often I was stumbling and collapsing to the ground. I could feel my guide pulling on the rope, and this time I pulled back.

"Andale, Andale! Nos vamos," he said to me with an infuriating smile, almost reveling in my exhaustion. If I had the energy, I would have slapped him.

It was at that moment that I realized I was in way over my head. I was too old for this shit, or at least too old to go at someone else's pace who was much younger than me (and a professional mountaineer). I had to respect my limits—and my age. So I unhooked the rope from my waist, turned off my headlamp, and lay down on the glacier and stared up at the moon. "I'm not going any farther," I announced. "I don't have to do this anymore" (giving voice to the mantra inside my head). "I just want to sit here and enjoy where I am. I want to look at the moon. I want to listen to the glacier. I earned this."

I've never felt more proud of myself than the choice *not* to summit the volcano. It felt like I was finally accepting, if not respecting, my limits as I age. It was an amazing experience for me precisely because I realized what I could do and what I couldn't. And this was a breakthrough for me as a therapist and a teacher.

I've mentioned earlier that I've always relied on my rather impressive memory. I could do three or four sessions in a row and not bother to write in the case files until the end of the day, recalling the conversations almost perfectly. I could see five clients in a row without a break or even the need to visit the bathroom. I could lead a two-day workshop and still have enough energy left over to go out and party all night. But those days are surely gone.

What I learned that night on the volcano is that there are, indeed, certain things I can't do any more. But, also, there are things I really don't want or need to do anymore.

From what I've been studying related to so-called "successful" or "adaptive" aging, there appears to be some consistent themes. Those who age well, especially those therapists who flourish during these "golden years," have developed a clear vision of their limitations as well as strengths and they make adjustments accordingly. They work within their capacity, rather than try to function as they did earlier in life. They are more selective in how they spend their time, more discerning with regard to the people with whom they socialize. With the acceptance of limited time left, they are inclined to prioritize those activities that are more satisfying, and they are less willing to engage in tasks that feel like a waste of time. The common mantra has evolved over time from, "I really don't want to do that," to "I don't *have* to do that anymore."

As for me? I say the right things. I even believe that it is a very good thing indeed to act my age, accept my limitations, and carefully measure realistic expectations for the future. But I'm not nearly done yet, if I have any choice in the matter. It feels like I have time to do one more thing, live one more life, adapt what I know and understand as a therapist to another new arena where I can be useful and do some good. And I'm not yet ready to throw in the towel and accept that I can't continue to seek out new, challenging, even strenuous adventures. What I did realize on the Ecuadorian volcano is that I now have more freedom than ever before to choose what I want to do and—just as important—to decide what I care not to do ever again.

Postscript and Full Disclosure

At the risk of being branded a hypocrite, I have a little confession to make. I actually haven't yet given up on my dream of summiting that damn volcano in Ecuador. For me, it is not about getting to the top of the mountain, but rather about seeing the spectacular crevasses, glaciers, ice caves, and views that would only be visible during daylight on the way down.

Okay, I'm probably lying. I really do want to see if I can make it. So I'm heading back to Ecuador as this book goes to press. I'm going to try some things differently, train harder, hire a different guide, adjust my equipment. But I'm also aware that I don't really need to get to the top; I just really want to enjoy the journey.

COMING TO TERMS WITH OUR OWN AGING

This project has been quite an adventure, given that it reflects our own lived experience and our own struggle to come to terms with who we are at this later stage of our lives. Both of us changed jobs this year. Both of us relocated to different geographic places. We have been in the process of reinventing ourselves, deciding what we want to do next and what we wish to do with the limited time we have left. This book obviously represents our own lived experience. We are fortunate to have picked the one area we feel most challenged and confused: what it means for us to age and how we are learning to cope with those changes. As this journey together with you comes to a close, regardless of your own age and stage of life, we wish to mention a few other things we learned along the way and how we have been impacted by this deep exploration into what it means to be old, as well as to be an older therapist.

We have been encouraged, most of all, to look *way* beyond what older clients present as their complaints in need of fixing. We certainly acknowledge that what brought them to therapy in the first place must be addressed, whether a family matter, an emotional disorder, a physical challenge, or some unresolved issue from the past. But, we also realize the importance of moving beyond those problems to focus on four specific domains that improve the quality of life. By way of summary, these are a few things that hit home.

1. There is a critical importance of encouraging older clients to remain physically active by recommending and structuring some sort of regular exercise program, whether that is stretching, yoga, walking, hiking, aerobics, or fitness classes.
2. We should prioritize the importance of remaining intellectually stimulated through some activity or endeavor that requires concentration, learning, and ongoing growth. Whether doing crossword puzzles, learning a language, taking classes, or writing one's memoirs, this is a key feature of minimizing cognitive loss to continue with lifelong learning.
3. Social interactions are so much a part of remaining actively engaged with the world.
4. Finally, we must recognize and honor one's limits and learn to adjust to realities in light of possible limitations.

When all is said and done, even with the seemingly frequent complaints about our losses and changes, we both enjoy being senior therapists and teachers. We have devoted more than 40 years each to this profession, and have accumulated so much experience and wisdom that allow us to understand things that seem so puzzling to others. Or perhaps we've just learned to accept certain things with equanimity and realize which battles we can truly fight with courage and commitment.

It feels wonderful to look back on our professional lives and know we have made a difference. We feel fortunate to have learned so much from our clients and students. We recognize honestly that we have lost a step or two, but we also acknowledge that this last stage of life brings with it so much unexpected joy and wisdom. Poet William Wordsworth remarked that life is divided into three types of consciousness: "that which was, which is, and which will be." He advised that we must learn from the past to help us function optimally in the present. And such focus on the present, on the precious moments each of us are granted every day, allows us to live more passionately and productively in the present, no matter how our days may be numbered.

REFERENCES

Abraham, K. (1919). The applicability of psycho-analytic treatment to patients at an advanced age. In *Selected Papers* (pp. 312–317). London: Hogarth Press.

Adelman, R. D., Tmanova, L. L., Delgado, D., Dion S., & Lachs, M. S. (2014). Caregiver burden: A clinical review. *Journal of the American Medical Association, 311*(10), 1052–1060.

Administration of Aging. (2011). *Census data and population estimates*. Washington, DC: Department of Health and Human Services.

Agronin, M. E. (2010). *Therapy with older adults: Key strategies for success*. New York: W. W. Norton.

American Psychological Association. (2014). Guidelines for psychological practice with older adults. *American Psychologist, 69*(1), 34–65.

Ameriprise Financial Survey. (2015). *The health and wealth connection in retirement*.

Anderson, E., & Johnson, S. (2010). Older people and their significant systems: Meeting with families and networks. In G. Fredman, E. Anderson, & J. Stott (Eds.), *Being with older people: A systemic approach* (pp. 113–138). London: Karnac.

Ansbacher, H. L., & Ansbacher, R. R. (Eds.). (1956). *The individual psychology of Alfred Adler: A systematic presentation in selections from his writings*. New York: Basic Books.

Ansbacher, H. L., & Ansbacher, R. R. (Eds.). (1962). *The individual psychology of Alfred Adler: A systematic presentation in selections from his writings*. New York: Harper Torchbooks.

Arnold, M. (2008). Polypharmacy and older adults: A role for psychology and psychologists. *Professional Psychology: Research and Practice, 39*(3), 283–289.

Aronson, K., & Weiner, M. B. (2007). *Aging parents, aging children*. Lanham, MD: Rowman & Littlefield.

Atkin, S., & Atkin, A. (1992). On being old (a psychiatrist's new world). In G. H. Pollock (Ed.), *How psychiatrists look at aging* (pp. 1–24). Madison, CT: International Universities Press.

Atkins, D., & Lowenthal, D. (2004). The lived experiences of psychotherapists working with older clients: An heuristic study. *British Journal of Guidance and Counselling, 32*(4), 499–505.

Baltes, P. B., Lindenberger, U., & Staudinger, U. M. (1998). Life-span theory in developmental psychology. In W. Damon & R. M. Lerner (Eds.), *Handbook of Child Psychology* (5th ed.), (pp. 1029–1143). New York: Wiley.

Bastowrous, M. (2013). Caregiver burden: A critical discussion. *International Journal of Nursing Studies, 50*, 431–441.

Bergner, R. M. (2007). Therapeutic storytelling revisited. *American Journal of Psychotherapy, 61*(2), 149–162.

Bermann, A. (2009). Reflections on aging, psychotherapy, and spiritual practice. *Women and Therapy, 32*, 267–274.
Berthelsdorf, S. (1992). Perspective at seventy-seven of prejudice, conflict, and aloneness. In G. H. Pollock (Ed.), *How psychiatrists look at aging* (pp. 55–68). Madison, CT: International Universities Press.
Bolgar, H. (2006). Film interview, from *The Beauty of Aging* [Online]. Available: http://www.beautyofaging.com/hedda-bolgar.html. Accessed March 8, 2014.
Bonnano, G. A., Wortman, C. B., & Nesse, R. M. (2004). Prospective patterns of resilience and maladjustment during widowhood. *Psychology & Aging, 19*(2), 260–271.
Borglin, G., Edberg, A. K., & Hallberg, I. R. (2005). The experience of quality of life among older people. *Journal of Aging Studies, 19*, 201–220.
Bormans, L. (Ed.). (2010). *The world book of happiness*. Singapore: Page One.
Brandtstedter, J. (1990). Tenacious goal pursuit and flexible goal adjustment: Explication and age-related analysis of assimilative and accommodative strategies of coping. *Psychology and Aging, 5*, 58–67.
Brenoff, A. (2014). 10 Things to let go of when you hit 50 [Online]. *Huffington Post*, January 17. Available: http://www.huffingtonpost.com/2014/01/17/things-to-let-go-of_n_4557231.html Accessed March 12, 2014.
Brickman, A. M., & Stern, Y. (2009). Aging and memory in humans. In L. R. Squire (Ed.), *Encyclopedia of Neuroscience*. New York: Academic Press.
Brody, J. E. (2007, November 27). A common casualty of old age: The will to live. *New York Times*, p. D7.
Bruce, E. (1999). Holding onto the story: Older people, narrative, and dementia. Roberts, G. (1999). Introduction: A story of stories. In G. Roberts & J. Holmes (Eds.), *Healing stories: Narrative in psychiatry and psychotherapy* (pp. 181–205). New York: Oxford University Press.
Bugental, J. (1985). *The art of the psychotherapist*. New York: Random House.
Burns, G. W. (Ed.). (2007). *Healing with stories: Your casebook for using therapeutic metaphors*. New York: Wiley.
Butler, R. (1963). The live review: An interpretation of reminiscence in the aged. *Psychiatry, 26*, 65–76.
Butler, R. (1974) Successful aging and the role of life review. *Journal of the American Geriatric Society, 22*, 529–535.
Butler, R. (2008). *The longevity revolution: The benefits and challenges of living a long life*. New York: Public Affairs.
Calhoun, L. G., & Tedeschi, R. G. (2013). *Posttraumatic growth in clinical practice*. New York: Routledge.
Carstensen, L. L. (2011). *A long bright future: Happiness, health, and financial security in an age of increased longevity*. New York: Public Affairs.
Carstensen, L. L., & Hartel, C. R. (Eds.). (2006). *When I'm 64*. Washington, DC: National Academies Press.
Charles, S. T., & Cartensen, L. L. (2010). Social and emotional aging. *Annual Review of Psychology, 61*, 383–409.
Charon, R. (2001). Narrative medicine: A model for empathy, reflection, profession, and trust. *Journal of the American Medical Association*.
Charon, R. (2006). *Narrative medicine: Honoring the stories of illness*. New York: Oxford University Press.
Chessick, R. D. (2013). Special problems for the elderly psychoanalyst in the psychoanalytic process. *Journal of the American Psychoanalytic Association, 61*, 67–92.

Chonody, J. M., Webb, S. N., Ranzjin, R., & Bryan, J. (2014). Working with older adults: Predictors of attitudes towards aging in psychology and social work students, faculty, and practitioners. *Australian Psychologist, 49*, 374–383.
Clower, V. L. (1992). Aging in a mirror. In G. H. Pollock (Ed.), *How psychiatrists look at aging* (pp. 69–84). Madison, CT: International Universities Press.
Cohen, G. D. (2005). *The mature mind: The positive power of the aging brain.* New York: Basic Books.
Cohen, G. D. (2006). Research on creativity and aging: The positive impact of the arts on health and illness. *Generations, 30*(1), 7–15.
Cooney, C., Howard, R., & Lawlor, B. (2006). Abuse of vulnerable people with dementia by their careers: Can we identify those most at risk? *International Journal of Geriatric Psychiatry, 21*, 564–571.
Coppola, K. M., & Trotman, F. K. (2002). Dying and death: Decisions at the end of life. In F. K. Trotman & C. M. Brody (Eds.), *Psychotherapy and counseling with older women: Cross-cultural, family, and end-of-life issues* (pp. 221–238). New York: Springer.
Crose, R. G. (2002). A woman's aging body: Friend or foe? In F. K. Trotman & C. M. Brody (Eds.), *Psychotherapy and counseling with older women: Cross-cultural, family, and end-of-life issues* (pp. 17–40). New York: Springer.
Cruikshank, M. (2009). *Learning to be old: Gender, culture, and aging* (2nd ed.). New York: Rowman & Littlefield.
Dans, P. E. (2002). The use of pejorative terms to describe patients: "Dirtball" revisted. *Baylor Medical Center Proceedings, 15*(1), 26–30.
Dening, T., & Thomas, A. (Eds.). (2013). *Oxford textbook of old age psychiatry.* New York: Oxford University Press.
De Shazer, S. (1985). *Keys to solution in brief therapy.* New York: W. W. Norton.
Diener, E. (Ed.). (2009). *The science of well-being.* New York: Springer.
Dittman, M. (2003). Fighting ageism. *APA Monitor, 43*(5), 50.
Dockendorff, D. C. T. (2014). Healthy ways of coping with losses related to the aging process. *Educational Gerontology, 40*, 363–384.
Dolittle, H. (1956). *Tribute to Freud.* New York: Pantheon.
Donlon, M. M., Ashman, O., & Levy, B. R. (2005). Re-vision of older television characters: A stereotype awareness intervention. *Journal of Social Issues, 61*(2), 307–319.
Duarte, N. (2010). *Resonate: Present visual stories that transform audiences.* New York: Wiley.
Duffy, M. (1992). Challenges in geriatric psychotherapy. *Individual Psychology, 48*(4), 432–440.
Duhigg, C. (2012). *The power of habit.* New York: Random House.
Eckardt, M. H. (1992). Viewing my own aging: A personal journey of contemplation. In G. H. Pollock (Ed.), *How psychiatrists look at aging* (pp. 85–95). Madison, CT: International Universities Press.
Edmundson, M. (2007). *The death of Sigmund Freud: The legacy of his last days.* New York: Bloomsbury.
Ellin, A. (2013, April 22). How therapy can help in the golden years [Online]. *New York Times*. Available: http://well.blogs.nytimes.com/2013/04/22/how-therapy-can-help-in-the-golden-years/?_php=true&_type=blogs&_r=0. Accessed March 18, 2014.
Erikson, J., & Erikson, E. (1989). *The life cycle completed.* New York: W. W. Norton.
Fields, H. (2012). What is so good about growing old [Online]. *Smithsonian*, July–August. Available: http://www.smithsonianmag.com/science-nature/

what-is-so-good-about-growing-old-130839848/?no-ist. Accessed November 14, 2014.
Fieldsteel, N. D. (2011). The aging therapist. *Group*, 35(1), 11–16.
Flick, U., Garms-Homolova, V., & Rohnsch, G. (2012). "And mostly they have a need for sleeping pills": Physicians' views on treatment of sleep disorders with drugs in nursing homes. *Journal of Aging Studies*, 26, 484–494.
Fonagy, P. (2009). When analysts need to retire: The taboo of ageing in psychoanalysis. In B. Willock, R. C. Curtis, & L. C. Bohm (Eds.), *Taboo or not taboo? Forbidden thoughts, forbidden acts in psychoanalysis and psychotherapy* (pp. 209–227). London: Karnac.
Francis, D. R. (2002). Why do death rates decline? *NBER Digest*, March, 3.
Franke, T., Tong, C., Ashe, M. C., McKay, H., Sims-Gould, J., et al. (2013). The secrets of highly active older adults. *Journal of Aging Studies*, 27, 398–409.
Frankl, V. E. (1986). *The doctor and the soul*. New York: Vantage.
Frazer, D. W., Hinrichsen, G. A., & Jongsma, A. E. (2014). *The older adult psychotherapy treatment planner* (2nd ed.). New York: Wiley.
Fredman, G., Anderson, E., & Stott, J. (Eds.). (2010). *Being with older people: A systemic approach*. London: Karnac.
Fredman, G., & Rapaport, P. (2010). How do we begin? Working with older people and their significant systems. In G. Fredman, E. Anderson, & J. Stott (Eds.), *Being with older people: A systemic approach* (pp. 31–59). London: Karnac.
Freedman, M. (1999). *Prime time: How baby boomers will revolutionize retirement and transform America*. New York: Public Affairs.
Freeman, M. (2011). Narrative foreclosure in later life: Possibilities and limits. In G. Kenyon, E. Bohlmeijer, & W. L. Randall (Eds.), *Storying later live: Issues, investigations and interventions in narrative gerontology* (pp. 3–19). New York: Oxford University Press.
Freud, S. (1905/1953). *On psychotherapy. Standard edition* (Vol. 7, p. 264). London: Hogarth Press.
Freud, S. (1927). Some psychological consequences of the anatomic distinction between the sexes. *Journal of Psycho-Analysis*, 8, 133–142.
Friedman, H. S., & Martin, L. R. (2012). *The longevity project*. New York: Plume.
Fry, P. S. (2000). Religious involvement, spirituality, and personal meaning for life: Existential predictors of psychological well-being in community-residing and institutional care elders. *Aging and Mental Health*, 4, 375–387.
Fung, H. H. (2013). Aging in culture. *The Gerontologist*, 53(3), 369–377.
Gardyn, R. (2002). Retirement redefined. *American Demographies, November*, 52
Gawande, A. (2014, March 25). The way we age now [Online]. *The New Yorker* Available: http://www.newyorker.com/reporting/2007/04/30/070430fa_fact_gawande. Accessed March 25, 2014.
Gay, P. (1971). *Freud: A life for our time*. New York: W. W. Norton.
Geller, J. D. (2014). Adult development and the transformative powers of psychotherapy. *Journal of Clinical Psychology*, 70(8), 768–779.
Gergen, M. M. (2009). Framing lives: Therapy with women of a "certain age." *Women and Therapy*, 32, 252–266.
Gilleard, C., & Higgs, P. (2007). The third age and baby boomers: Two approaches to the social structuring of later life. *International Journal of Aging and Later Life*, 2, 13–30.
Gillick, M. R. (2006). *The denial of aging*. Cambridge, MA: Harvard University Press.
Glicken, M. D. (2009). *Evidence-based counseling and psychotherapy for an aging population*. New York: Academic Press.

Glisky, E. L. (2007). Changes in cognitive function in human aging. In D. R. Riddle (Ed.), *Brain aging: Models, methods, and mechanisms* (pp. 1–15). Boca Raton, FL: CRC Press.
Goldberg, E. (2005). *The wisdom paradox: How your mind can grow stronger as your brain grows older.* New York: Free Press.
Gomberg, E. S. (1996). Alcohol and drugs. In J. E. Birren (Ed.), *Encyclopedia of Gerontology.* New York: Academic Press.
Gottschall, J. (2012). *The storytelling animal: How stories make us human.* New York: Houghton Mifflin.
Gregoire, C. (2014, March 3). 18 Things highly creative people do differently [Online]. *Huffington Post.* Available: http://www.huffingtonpost.com/2014/03/04/creativity-habits_n_4859769.html?view=print&comm_ref=false. Accessed March 4, 2014.
Gullette, M. M. (2011). *Agewise: Fighting the new ageism in America.* Chicago, IL: University of Chicago Press.
Gum, A., King-Kallimanis, B., & Kohn, R. (2009). Prevalence of mood, anxiety, and substance-abuse disorders for older Americans in the National Comorbidity Survey Replication. *American Journal of Geriatric Psychiatry, 17*(9), 769–781.
Guy, J. D., Stark, M. J., Poelstra, P., & Souder, J. K. (1987). Psychotherapist retirement and age-related impairment: Results of a national survey. *Psychotherapy, 24,* 816–820.
Hall, S. S. (2001, March 11). Prescription for profit. *New York Times,* pp. 40–45.
Hanna, G. P. (2013). The central role of creativity in aging. *Journal of Art for Life, 4*(1), 1–15.
Hawkes, K., & Coxworth, J. E. (2013). Grandmothers and the evolution of human longevity: A review of findings and future directions. *Evolutionary Anthropology, 22,* 294–302.
Haybron, D. M. (2008). *The pursuit of unhappiness: The elusive psychology of well-being.* New York: Oxford University Press.
Hazan, H. (1994). *Old age: Construction and deconstructions.* New York: Oxford University Press.
Hazan, H. (2011). From ageless self to selfless age: Toward a theoretical turn in gerontological understanding. In L. W. Poon & J. Cohen-Mansfield (Eds.), *Understanding well-being in the oldest old* (pp. 11–26). New York: Cambridge University Press.
Hepple, J. (2004). Psychotherapies with older people: An overview. *Advances in Psychiatric Treatment, 10,* 371–377.
Hicks, M. (2012). Private practice: Musings of an aging therapist [Online]. *National Association of Social Workers.* Available: http://naswil.org/news/chapter-news/featured/private-practice-musings-of-an-aging-therapist/. Accessed March 18, 2014.
Hildebrand, H. P. (1990). Towards a psychodynamic understanding of later life. In M. Bergener & S. I. Finkel (Eds.), *Clinical and scientific psychogeriatrics.* New York: Springer.
Hill, R. D. (2005). *Positive aging.* New York: W. W. Norton.
Hillman, J. (1990). *Suicide and the soul.* Dallas, TX: Spring.
Hinrichsen, G. A., & Clougherty, K. F. (2006). *Interpersonal psychotherapy for depressed older adults.* Washington, DC: American Psychological Association.
Holliday S. G., & Chandler, M. J. (1986). Wisdom: Explorations in adult competence. In J. A. Meacham (Ed.), *Contributions to human development* (Vol. 17), (pp. 1–96). Basil, Switzerland: Karger.
Hurwitz, M. H. (1992). A psychoanalyst retires. In G. H. Pollock (Ed.), *How psychiatrists look at aging* (pp. 97–108). Madison, CT: International Universities Press.

Hyer, L, Yeager, C. A., & Scott, C. V. (2011). Late-life psychotherapy: Challenges and opportunities. In L. W. Poon & J. Cohen-Mansfield (Eds.), *Understanding well-being in the oldest old* (pp. 332–363). New York: Cambridge University Press.

Ingemark, C. A. (Ed.). (2013). *Therapeutic uses of storytelling*. Lund, Sweden: Nordic Academic Press.

Ionedes, N. S. (1979). Adlerian psychotherapy in practice: The case of Mr. and Mrs. T. *Journal of Individual Psychology, 35*(1), 70–78.

Ionedes, N. S. (1992). A therapy program for Alzheimer's disease: An Adlerian orientation. *Individual Psychology, 48*(4), 413–418.

Irving, D. (2013). Gerontology: A glance at the adult aging population. *Counseling Today, September*, 28–29.

Jamieson, J. P., Nock, M. K., & Mendes, W. B. (2012). Mind over matter: Reappraising arousal improves cardiovascular and cognitive responses to stress. *Journal of Experimental Psychology, 141*(3), 417–422.

Jeste, D. V., & Oswald, A. J. (2014). Individual and societal wisdom: Explaining the paradox of human aging and high well-being. *Psychiatry, 77*(4), 317–330.

Joseph, S. (2011). *What doesn't kill us: The new psychology of posttraumatic growth*. New York: Basic Books.

Kahanna, R. (2005, November 27). Katrina's aftermath. *Houston Chronicle*.

Kalanithi, P. (2015). Before I go. *Stanford medicine*, Spring.

Kampfe, C. M. (2014). *Counseling older people: Opportunities and challenges*. Alexandria, VA: ACA Press.

Kashdan, T. B. (2008, August 19). Why are we afraid of having regrets [Online]? *Psychology Today*. Available: https://www.psychologytoday.com/blog/curious/201008/why-are-we-afraid-having-regrets.

Keller, A., Litzelman, K., Wisk, L. E., Maddox, T., Cheng, E. R., Creswell, P. D., & Witt, W. P. (2012). Does the perception that stress affects health matter? The association with health and mortality. *Health Psychology, 31*(5), 677–684.

Kennedy, G. J., & Tannenbaum, S. (2000). Psychotherapy with aging adults. *American Journal of Psychotherapy, 54*, 386–407.

Kenyon, G., Bohlmeijer, E., & Randall, W. L. (Eds.). (2011). *Storying later live: Issues, investigations and interventions in narrative gerontology*. New York: Oxford University Press.

Kirkpatrick, M. (1992). Aging, like a woman. In G. H. Pollock (Ed.), *How psychiatrists look at aging* (pp. 141–147). Madison, CT: International Universities Press.

Kirschenbaum, H. (2008). *Life and work of Carl Rogers*. Alexandria, VA: American Counseling Association.

Kluger, J. (2013, September 23). The art of living. *Time*, 45–50.

Knight, B. G. (2004). *Psychotherapy with older adults* (3rd ed.). Thousand Oaks, CA: Sage.

Knight, B. G., & Sayegh, P. (2010). Cultural values and caregiving: The updated sociocultural stress and coping model. *Journal of Gerontology, 65*, 5–13.

Korkki, P. (2014, March 12). The science of older and wiser [Online]. *New York Times*. Available: http://www.nytimes.com/2014/03/13/business/retirementspecial/the-science-of-older-and-wiser.html?_r=0. Accessed April 19, 2014.

Kottler, J. A. (2010). *The assassin and the therapist: An exploration of truth in psychotherapy and in life*. New York: Routledge.

Kottler, J. A. (2015). *Stories we've heard, stories we've told: Life-changing narratives in therapy and everyday life*. New York: Oxford University Press.

Kottler, J. A., & Carlson, J. (2002). *Bad therapy: Master therapists share their worst failures*. New York: Brunner/Routledge.

Kottler, J. A., & Carlson, J. (2003). *The mummy at the dining room table: Eminent therapists reveal their most unusual cases and what they teach us about human behavior.* San Francisco: Jossey-Bass.

Kottler, J. A., & Carlson, J. (2006). *The client who changed me: Stories of therapist personal transformation.* New York: Brunner/Routledge.

Kottler, J. A., & Carlson, J. (2007). *Moved by the spirit: Discovery and transformation in the lives of leaders.* Atascadero, CA: Impact.

Kottler, J. A., & Carlson, J. (2008). *Their finest hour: Master therapists share their greatest success stories* (2nd ed.). Bethel, CT: Crown Publishing.

Kottler, J. A., & Carlson, J. (2009). *Creative breakthroughs in therapy: Tales of transformation and astonishment.* New York: Wiley

Kottler, J. A., & Carlson, J. (2011). *Duped: Lies and deception in psychotherapy.* New York: Routledge.

Kottler, J. A., & Carlson, J. (2015). *On being a master therapist: Practicing what we preach.* New York: Wiley.

Kottler, J. A., Carlson, J., & Keeney, B. (2004). *An American shaman: An odyssey of ancient healing traditions.* New York: Brunner/Routledge.

Kottler, J. A., Englar-Carlson, M., & Carlson, J. (Eds.). (2013). *Helping beyond the 50 minute hour: Therapists involved in meaningful social action.* New York: Routledge.

Kottler, J. A., & Marriner, M. (2009). *Changing people's lives while transforming your own: Paths to social justice and global human rights.* New York: Wiley.

Kraus, G. (2012). Psychotherapy with older adults: Unjustified fears, unrecognized rewards [Online]. *Psychotherapy.net.* Available: https://www.psychotherapy.net/article/geriatric-psychotherapy. Accessed March 8, 2014.

Kray, L. J., George, L. G., Liljenquist, K. A., Galinsky, A. D., Tetlock, P. E., & Roese, N. J. (2010). From what might have been to what must have been: Counterfactual thinking creates meaning. *Journal of Personality and Social Psychology, 98,* 106–118.

Laidlaw, K., & Pachana, N. A. (2009). Aging, mental health, and demographic change: Challenges for psychotherapists. *Professional Psychology: Research and Practice, 40*(6), 601–608.

Langle, A., & Probst, C. (2000). Existential questions of the elderly. *International Medical Journal,* 7(5), 193–196.

Lawrence-Lightfoot, S. (2009). *The third chapter: Passion, risk, and adventure in the 25 years after 50.* New York: Sara Crighton Books.

Leavy, S. A. (2011). The last of life: Psychological reflections on old age and death. *The Psychoanalytic Quarterly, 80*(3), 699–715.

Lee, Y. S. (2009). Measures of student attitudes on aging. *2,* 121–134.

Leigland, L. A., Schulz, L. E., & Jankowsky, J. S. (2004). Age related changes in emotional memory. *Neurobiological Aging, 25*(8), 1117–1124.

Levine, M. (2004, June 1). Tell your doctor all your problems, but keep it less than a minute [Online]. *New York Times.* Available: http://www.nytimes.com/2004/06/01/health/tell-the-doctor-all-your-problems-but-keep-it-to-less-than-a-minute.html?pagewanted=all&src=pm.

Levy, B. R., Slade, M. D., Kunkel, S. R., & Kasl, S. V. (2002). Longevity increased by positive self-perceptions of aging. *Journal of Personality and Social Psychology, 83,* 261–270.

Levy, B. R., Slade, M. D., Murphy, T. E., & Gill, T. M. (2012). Association between positive age stereotypes and recovery from disability in older persons. *Journal of the American Medical Association, 308*(19), 1972–1973.

Lewis, A. M. (2014). Terror management theory applied clinically: Implications for existential–integrative psychotherapy. *Death Studies, 38*, 412–417.

Liebenberg, B. (2011). How old is your therapist? *Group, 35*(1), 41–44.

Loe, M. (2011). *Aging our way: Independent elders, independent lives*. New York: Oxford University Press.

Loeb, E. (2009). The therapist at 60, the patient at 60: Challenges for psychotherapy. *Women and Therapy, 32*, 186–201.

Lopez, S. (2011, October 2). At age 102, therapist is too busy to stop working [Online]. *Los Angeles Times*. Available: http://articles.latimes.com/2011/oct/02/local/la-me-1002-lopez-bolgar-20111002. Accessed March 8, 2014.

Lun, M. W. A. (2011). Student knowledge and attitudes toward older people and their impact on pursuing aging careers. *Educational Gerontology, 37*(1), 1–11.

Lyons, I. (2009). *Public perceptions of older people and aging: A literature review*. Dublin, Ireland: National Centre for the Protection of Older People.

Lyubomirsky, S. (2013). *The myths of happiness*. New York: Penguin.

Mackenzie, A., & Greenwood, N. (2012). Positive experiences of caregiving in stroke: A systematic review. *Disability and Rehabilitation, 34*(17), 1413–1422.

MacKinlay, E. (2014). Baby boomers ageing well? Challenges in the search for meaning in later life. *Journal of Religion, Spirituality, and Aging, 26*, 109–121.

Maijala, E. L., Uusiautti, S., & Maatta, K. (2013). Grandparental love: A challenge or a richness? *Early Child Development and Care, 183*(5), 627–642.

Martin, L. J. (1944). *Handbook for old age counselors*. San Francisco, CA: Geetz.

Martin, P., Da Rosa, G., & Poon, L. W. (2011). The impact of life events on the oldest old. In L. W. Poon & J. Cohen-Mansfield (Eds.), *Understanding well-being in the oldest old* (pp. 96–110). New York: Cambridge University Press.

Masoro, E. J., & Austad, S. N. (Eds.). (2010). *Handbook of the biology of aging* (7th ed.). San Diego, CA: Academic Press.

May, R. (1967). *Existential psychology*. Toronto, Canada: CBC.

McKee, P., & Barber, C. (1999). On defining wisdom. *International Journal of Aging and Human Development, 49*(2), 149–164.

Mehl-Madrona, L. (2007). *Narrative medicine: The use of history and story in the healing*. Rochester, VT: Bear and Company.

Mehl-Madrona, L. (2010). *Healing the mind through the power of story*. Rochester, VT: Bear and Company.

Michalski, D., & Kohut, J. (2008). *APA survey of psychology health service providers*. Washington, DC: American Psychological Association.

Milton, A., & Hansen, E. (2010). Moving from problems to possibilities with older people. In G. Fredman, E. Anderson, & J. Stott (Eds.), *Being with older people: A systemic approach* (pp. 161–180). London: Karnac.

Molinari, V. (1999) Using reminiscence and life review as natural therapeutic strategies in group therapy. In M. Duffy (Ed.), *Handbook of counseling and psychotherapy with older adults* (pp. 154–165). New York: John Wiley.

Molnar, M. (Ed.). (1992). *The diary of Sigmund Freud*. New York: Scribners.

Moody, H. R., & Sasser, J. R. (2015). *Aging: Concepts and controversies* (8th ed.). Thousand Oaks, CA: Sage.

Moraglia, G. (2004). On facing death: Views of some prominent psychologists. *Journal of Humanistic Psychology, 44*(3), 337–357.

Munn, J. C., Zimmerman, S., Hanson, L. C., Williams, C. S., Sloane, P. D., Clipp, E. C., Tulsky, J. A., & Steinhauser, K. E. (2007). Measuring the quality of dying in long-term care. *Journal of the American Geriatrics Society, 55*(9), 1371–1379.

Musaiger, A. O., & D'Souza, R. (2009). Role of age and gender in the perception of aging. *Archives of Gerontology and Geriatrics, 48*(1), 50–57.
Narrow, W. E., Rae, D. S., Robins, L. N., & Regier, D. A. (2002). Revisted prevalence based estimates of mental disorders in the United States. *Archives of General Psychiatry, 59*, 115–123.
National Association of Social Workers. (2006). *Who are licensed social workers* [Online]? Available: http://workforce.socialworkers.org/studies/supplemental/supplement_ch2.pdf.
National Council on Aging (2013). *United States of aging survey* [Online]. Available: https://www.ncoa.org/news/usoa-survey/.
Neighmond, P. (2014). A coping plan to help fend off depression from vision loss [Online]. *National Public Radio*. Available: http://www.npr.org/blogs/health/2014/08/11/338592866/a-coping-plan-can-help-fend-off-depression-from-vision-loss
Neimeyer, R. A. (2004). Fostering posttraumatic growth: A narrative contribution. *Psychological Inquiry, 15*, 53–59.
Nelson, T. D. (2005). Ageism: Prejudice against our feared future self. *Journal of Social Issues, 61*, 207–221.
O'Connell, W. E. (1992). The public practice of Adlerian wisdom with the elderly. *Individual Psychology, 48*(4), 441–450.
O'Hanlon, B. (1993). *A brief guide to brief therapy*. New York: W. W. Norton.
Olshansky, J. (2011). Aging of U.S. presidents. *Journal of the American Medical Association, 306*(21), 2328–2329.
Oritz, L., & Langer, L. (2002). Assessment of spirituality and religion in later life: Acknowledging clients' needs and personal resources. *Journal of Gerontological Social Work, 37*, 5–21.
Palmore, E. (2001). The ageism survey: First findings. *The Gerontologist, 41*(5), 572–575.
Patterson, M. C., & Perlstein, S. (2011). Good for the heart, good for the soul: The creative arts and brain health in later life. *Generations, 35*(2), 27–36.
Pennington, S. (2009). Aging with my clients. *Women and Therapy, 32*, 202–208.
Pilling, D. (2003, August 7). Japan could export surplus centenarians. *Financial Times*, p. 1.
Pipher, M. (1999). *Another country*. New York: Riverhead.
Poon, L. W., & J. Cohen-Mansfield, J. (Eds.). (2011). *Understanding well-being in the oldest old*. New York: Cambridge University Press.
Post, S. G. (2005). Altruism, happiness, and health: It's good to be good. *International Journal of Behavioral Medicine, 12*(2), 66–77.
Qualls, S. H., & Williams, A. A. (2012). *Caregiver family therapy: Empowering families to meet the challenges of aging*. Washington, DC: APA Books.
Quill, T. E. (2000). Initiating end-of-life discussions with seriously ill patients. *Journal of the American Medical Association, 285*, 2506.
Rando, T. K. (2000). *Clinical dimensions of anticipatory mourning: Theory and practice in working with the dying and their loved ones, and their caregivers*. Champaign, IL: Research Press.
Richman, J. (2006). The role of psychotherapy and humor for death anxiety, death wishes, and aging. *Omega, 54*(1), 41–51.
Riffin, C., Ong, A. D., & Bergman, C. S. (2014). Positive emotions and health in adulthood and later life. In P. Verhaeghen & C. Hertzog (Eds.), *The Oxford handbook of emotion, social cognition, and problem solving in adulthood* (pp. 115–127). New York: Oxford University Press.
Roese, N. J. (2005). *If only: How to turn regret into opportunity*. New York: Broadway Books.
Rogers, C. R. (1980a). *A way of being*. Boston, MA: Houghton Mifflin.

Rogers, C. R. (1980b). Growing old—or older and growing. *Journal of Humanistic Psychology, 20*(4), 5–16.
Roseborough, D. J., Luptak, M., McLeod, J., & Bradshaw, W. (2013). Effectiveness of psychodynamic psychotherapy with older adults: A longitudinal study. *Clinical Gerontologist, 36*, 1–16.
Rosen, D. C., Miller, A. B., Nakash, O., Halpern, L., & Algeria, M. (2012). Interpersonal complementarity in the mental health intake: A mixed-methods study. *Journal of Counseling Psychology, 59*(2), 185–196.
Saffrey, C., Summerville, A., & Roese, N. J. (2008). Praise for regret: People value regret above other negative emotions. *Motivation and Emotion, 32*(1), 46–54.
Salthouse, T. A. (2012). Consequences of age-related cognitive declines. *Annual Review of Psychology, 63*, 201–226.
Sands, S. H. (2009). Less time ahead, more behind: Being a psychotherapist in the last third of life. *Women and Therapy, 32*, 158–169.
Scalmati, A., & Kennedy, G. J. (2009). Psychotherapy as end-of-life care: Special considerations for the older patient. *Psychiatric Annals, 39*(9), 833–837.
Schachter, J., Kachele, H. & Schachter, J. S. (2014). Psychotherapeutic/psychoanalytic treatment of the elderly. *Psychodynamic Psychiatry, 42*(1), 51–64.
Schafe, K. W. (2012). *Developmental influences on adult intelligence* (2nd ed.). New York: Oxford University Press.
Scott-Maxwell, F. (1968). *The measure of my days*. New York: Penguin.
Scully, J. H., & Wilk, J. E. (2003). Selected characteristics and data of psychiatrists in the United States [Online]. *Academic Psychiatry, 27*(4). Available: http://ap.psychiatryonline.org/article.aspx?articleID=47874.
Seaburn, D. (2013). More more time. *Psychotherapy Networker, September/October*, 79–80.
Seery, M. D., Holman, E. A., & Silver, R. C. (2010). Whatever does not kill us: Cumulative lifetime adversity, vulnerability, and resilience. *Journal of Personality and Social Psychology, 99*, 1025–1041.
Seligman, M. (2011). *Flourish: A visionary new understanding of happiness and well-being*. New York: Free Press.
Seligman, M., & Csikszentmihalyi, M. (2000). Positive psychology: An introduction. *American Psychologist, 55*, 5–14.
Settlage, C. F. (1996). Transcending old age. *International Journal of Psychoanalysis, 77*, 547–564.
Shiplett, J. L. (1996). *A glass full of tears*. Writer's World Press.
Shmotkin, D. (2005). Happiness in the face of adversity: Reformulating the dynamic and modular bases of subjective well-being. *Review of General Psychology, 9*, 291–325.
Shmotkin, D. (2011). The pursuit of happiness: Alternative conceptions of subjective well-being. In L. W. Poon & J. Cohen-Mansfield (Eds.), *Understanding well-being in the oldest old* (pp. 27–45). New York: Cambridge University Press.
Solis, J., & Brink, T. L. (1992). Adlerian approaches in geriatric psychotherapy: Case of an American widow. *Individual Psychology, 48*(4), 419–426.
Sorrell, J. M. (2014). Moving beyond caregiver burden. *Journal of Psychosocial Nursing, 52*(3), 15–18.
Sperber, M. (1974). *Masks of loneliness: Alfred Adler in perspective*. New York: Macmillan.
Sperry, L. (1992). Psychotherapy systems: An Adlerian integration with implication for older adults. *Individual Psychology, 48*(4), 451–461.
Sternberg, R. (Ed.). (1990). *Wisdom: Its nature, origins, and development*. New York: Cambridge University Press.

Stoller, R. J. (1992). Blessed denial: Or how, by aging, I (almost) conquered reality. In G. H. Pollock (Ed.), *How psychiatrists look at aging* (pp. 219–232). Madison, CT: International Universities Press.

Stuart-Hamilton, I. (2012). *The psychology of ageing: An introduction* (5th ed.). London: Jessica Kingsley.

Suri, R. (2010). Working with the elderly: An existential–humanistic approach. *Journal of Humanistic Psychology, 50*(2), 175–186.

Szalavitz, M. (2011, December 7). Why American presidents (and some Oscar winners) live longer [Online]. *Time*. Available: http://healthland.time.com/2011/12/07/why-american-presidents-and-some-oscar-winners-live-longer/. Accessed March 4, 2014.

Tallmer, M. (1992). The aging therapist. *Psychoanalytic Review, 79*(3), 388–404.

Tan, S. (2011). Wise up: The latest on aging and memory [Online]. *Psychology Today*. Available: http://www.psychologytoday.com/blog/wise/201101/myths-aging. Accessed November 20, 2013.

Tan, P. P., Zhang, N. H., & Fan, L. (2004). Students' attitudes toward the elderly in the People's Republic of China. *Educational Gerontology, 30*(4), 305–314.

Taylor, P. (Ed.). (2009). Growing old in America: Expectations versus reality [Online]. *Pew Research social and demographic trends: Overview and executive summary*. Available: http://www.pewsocialtrends.org/2009/06/29/growing-old-in-america-expectations-vs-reality/. Accessed March 11, 2014.

Thompson, A. (1991). Freud's pessimism, the death instinct, and the theme of disintegration in "Analysis terminable and interminable." *International Review of Psychoanalysis, 18*, 165–179.

Thornton, J. E. (2002). Myths of aging or ageist stereotypes. *Educational Gerontology, 28*, 301–312.

Tomko, J. K., & Munley, P. H. (2013). Predicting counseling psychologists attitudes and clinical judgments with respect to older adults. *Aging and Mental Health, 17*(2), 233–241.

Tornstam, L. (2005). *Gerotranscendence: A developmental theory of positive aging*. New York: Springer.

Trotman, F. K., & Brody, C. M. (2002a). Cross-cultural perspectives: Grandmothers. In F. K. Trotman & C. M. Brody (Eds.), *Psychotherapy and counseling with older women: Cross-cultural, family, and end-of-life issues* (pp. 41–58). New York: Springer.

Trotman, F. K., & Brody, C. M. (Eds.). (2002b). *Psychotherapy and counseling with older women: Cross-cultural, family, and end-of-life issues*. New York: Springer.

Tsai, K. C. (2013). A review of the inquiry of creativity in older adults in journals. *British Journal of Education, 1*(2), 20–28.

Vaillant, G. (2007). Aging well. *American Journal of Geriatric Psychiatry, 15*(3), 181–183.

Van Dussen, D. J., & Weaver, R. R. (2009). Undergraduate students perceptions and behaviors related to the aged and the aging process. *Educational Gerontology, 35*(1), 340–355.

Vaupel, M. (2010). Biodemography of human ageing. *Nature, 464*, 536–542.

Wass, H., & Neimeyer, R. A. (Eds.). (1995). *Dying: Finding the facts*. New York: Taylor and Francis.

Weiner, M. F. (1990). Older psychiatrists and their psychotherapy practice. *American Journal of Psychotherapy, XLIV*(1), 44–49.

Weiss, T. (2014). Personal transformation: Posttraumatic growth and gerotranscendence. *Journal of Humanistic Psychology, 54*(2), 203–226.

Weissman, M. M., Markowtiz, J. C., & Klerman, G. L. (2000). *Comprehensive guide to interpersonal psychotherapy*. New York: Basic Books.

White, M. (2000). *Reflections on narrative practice: Essays and interviews*. Adelaide: Dulich Centre Publications.

Wiles, J. L., & Jayasinha, R. (2013). Care for place: The contributions of older people make to their communities. *Journal of Aging Studies, 27*, 93–101.

Williams, G. C. (1957). Pleiotropy, natural selection, and the evolution of senescence. *Evolution, 11*(4), 398–411.

Wilson, I. B., Schoen, C., Neuman, P., Strollo, M. K., Rogers, W. H., Chang, H., & Safran, D. G. (2007). Physician–patient communication about prescription medication nonadherence: A 50-state study of America's seniors. *Journal of General Internal Medicine, 22*(1), 6–12.

Woodhead, E. L., Ivan, I. I., & Emery, E. E. (2013). Impact of older adults' experience with psychotherapy on treatment engagement. *Clinical Gerontologist, 36*, 260–273.

Wright, C. L. (2006, November 7). Changing directions and finding yourself. *New York Times*, p. 7.

Yalom, I. D. (1980). *Existential psychotherapy*. New York: Basic Books.

Yalom, I. D. (2005). *The Schopenhauer cure*. New York: HarperCollins.

Yalom, I. D. (2006). *The Schopenhauer cure*. New York: HarperPerennial.

Yalom, I. D. (2008). Staring at the sun: Overcoming the terror of death. *Humanistic Psychologist, 36*(3), 283–297.

Yalom, I. D. (2009). *Staring at the sun: Overcoming the terror of death*. San Francisco: Jossey-Bass.

Yalom, I. D. (2015). *Creatures of a day and other tales of psychotherapy*. New York: Basic Books.

Yang, J. A., Garis, J., Jackson, C., & McClure, R. (2009). Providing psychotherapy to older adults in home: Benefits, challenges, and decision-making guidelines. *Clinical Gerontologist, 32*, 333–346.

Zivian, M. T., Larsen, W., Knox, J. V., Gekoski, W. L., & Hatchette, V. (1992). Psychotherapy for the elderly: Psychotherapists' preferences. *Psychotherapy: Theory, Research, and Practice, 29*(4), 668–674.

Zolyniak, N., Schulte-Gocking, H., & Kraft, E. (2014). Neuroplasticity in aging: Implications for behavioral and lifestyle combined interventions. *Topics in Geriatric Rehabilitation, 30*(1), 15–17.

INDEX